Sticky Notes

✓ **HIPAA Compliant**
✓ **OSHA Compliant**

W0018853

Waterproof and Reusable
Wipe-Free Pages

Write directly onto any page of *Assess Notes* with a ballpoint pen. Wipe old entries off with an alcohol pad and reuse.

Look for our other
Davis's Notes titles

RNotes®: *Nurse's Clinical Pocket Guide, 2nd edition*
ISBN-10: 0-8036-1335-0 / ISBN-13: 978-0-8036-1335-5

LPN Notes: *Nurse's Clinical Pocket Guide, 2nd edition*
ISBN-10: 0-8036-1767-4 / ISBN-13: 978-0-8036-1767-4

NCLEX-RN® Notes: *Core Review & Exam Prep*
ISBN-10: 0-8036-1570-1 / ISBN-13: 978-0-8036-1570-0

PsychNotes: *Clinical Pocket Guide, 2nd edition*
ISBN-10: 0-8036-1853-0 / ISBN-13: 978-0-8036-1853-4

ECG Notes: *Interpretation and Management Guide*
ISBN-10: 0-8036-1347-4 / ISBN-13: 978-0-8036-1347-8

IV Therapy Notes: *Nurse's Clinical Pocket Guide*
ISBN-10: 0-8036-1288-5 / ISBN-13: 978-0-8036-1288-4

LabNotes: *Guide to Lab and Diagnostic Tests*
ISBN-10: 0-8036-1265-6 / ISBN-13: 978-0-8036-1265-5

MedNotes: *Nurse's Pharmacology Pocket Guide, 2nd edition*
ISBN-10: 0-8036-1531-0 / ISBN-13: 978-0-8036-1531-1

MedSurg Notes: *Nurse's Clinical Pocket Guide, 2nd edition*
ISBN-10: 0-8036-1868-9 / ISBN-13: 978-0-8036-1868-8

NutriNotes: *Nutrition & Diet Therapy Pocket Guide*
ISBN-10: 0-8036-1114-5 / ISBN-13: 978-0-8036-1114-6

OB Peds Women's Health Notes: *Nurse's Clinical Pocket Guide*
ISBN-10: 0-8036-1466-7 / ISBN-13: 978-0-8036-1466-6

*For a complete list of Davis's Notes and
other titles for health care providers,
visit www.fadavis.com*

Assess
Notes

Nursing Assessment & Diagnostic Reasoning

Marjory Gordon, PhD, RN, FAAN
Professor Emeritus,
Boston College School of Nursing

Purchase additional copies of this book
at your health science bookstore or
directly from F. A. Davis by shopping
online at www.fadavis.com or by calling
800-323-3555 (US) or 800-665-1148 (CAN)

A Davis's Notes Book

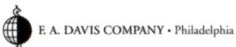

F. A. DAVIS COMPANY · Philadelphia

Publisher, Nursing: Joanne Patzek DaCunha, RN, MSN
Developmental Editor: William Welsh
Director of Content Development: Darlene D. Pedersen
Project Editor: Padraic J. Maroney
Manager of Art and Design: Carolyn O'Brien

Assessment and the Functional Health Patterns

Assessment is the collection and interpretation of information. It offers a glimpse into the perceptions, meanings, and logic patients use to organize and make sense of their world. Data are used in the three types of professional judgment within the nursing process:

- **Diagnostic judgment:** Identification of an actual or potential health problem.
- **Therapeutic judgment:** Decisions about intervention, outcome projection, and evaluation.
- **Ethical judgment:** Identification of an actual or potential moral problem.

Purpose of Assessment

The information gathered during an assessment is not merely collected and recorded. It is used to evaluate health status and to make a judgment about:

- Whether a problem or potential problem exists that requires nursing intervention.
- Status of a previously identified problem or condition in relation to projected outcomes.
- Strengths present in the situation, be it an individual, family, or community, that can be used to help solve problems.

These judgments represent reasoning, analysis, and information interpretation. The results are decisions about nursing diagnosis and intervention.

Assessment Standards

Assessment and diagnosis are included in the American Nurses Association's (2000) six Standards of Care and criteria for competent nursing practice. The standards are similar to the nursing process. Nurses use them for self-evaluation; consumers can use them to evaluate their nursing care; and lawyers use them to evaluate the quality of care and competency of the nurse in malpractice suits (Harkreader & Hogan, 2004, p. 215). The two standards related to assessment and diagnosis are:

- **Standard I:** The nurse collects health data systematically. The ongoing collection involves the patient, family and, when appropriate, other care providers.
- **Standard II:** The nurse analyzes assessment data in determining diagnoses. When possible, judgments are validated with the patient. Assessment data and diagnoses are documented and used in therapeutic decisions. (Excerpted from American Nurses Association [2000], with permission.)

Because assessment is the first phase of the nursing process, errors or omissions can affect all phases that follow.

Types of Assessment

Four types of assessment are used in nursing practice:

- **Emergency assessment:** Used in every encounter to complete a 2-7-second evaluation of the heart-lung-brain complex, including:
  - State of consciousness
  - Skin color
  - Posture
  - Activity
  - Facial expression
  - Speech
  - Pulse (if indicated)
  - Blood pressure (if indicated)
  - Respiration (if indicated)
- **Problem-focused assessment:** Used to evaluate the status of a previously diagnosed problem.
- **Time-lapse reassessment:** Used in clinic visits or in residential and long-term care when 3, 6, or 12 months have elapsed since the last assessment. It screens patterns and evaluates and evaluates previously identified nursing and medical diagnoses.
- **Admission assessment:** An admission assessment is the most complex type of assessment due to the minimal information initially available on a new patient. It involves assessing for a large amount of information and requires an organized approach regarding what to assess and how to proceed.

Because it is the most complex, the following discussion focuses on the admission assessment.

Admission Assessment

The information collected and the judgments made during the admission assessment are used in many ways. These extend from patient care to nurse staffing decisions and even to health statistics and nursing research. When patient care is the objective, the results of the admission assessment provide baseline information that can be used to project outcomes and measure change.

Accuracy is required at every level. For accuracy in clinical judgment, assessment needs to be systematic and deliberate.

■ **Systematic** means organized information collection and logical sequencing of questions.
■ **Deliberate** means assessment has purpose and direction. The basic information to be collected is clear.

Functional health patterns and the history and examination provide content and structure for the admission assessment.

Functional Health Patterns

Questions always arise about what information to collect, in what sequence, and how extensive the assessment should be. Functional health patterns provide:

■ Items to assess.
■ Structure for organizing assessment data.
■ Purpose and direction to health status evaluation and diagnosis.

The 11 functional health patterns for use with individuals, families, and communities are:

■ **Health perception–health management pattern:** Describes perceived pattern of health and well-being and how health is managed.
■ **Nutritional-metabolic pattern:** Describes the pattern of food and fluid consumption relative to metabolic need. Also included are pattern indicators of local nutrient supply.
■ **Elimination pattern:** Describes patterns of excretory function, including bowel, bladder, and skin excretory functions.
■ **Activity-exercise pattern:** Describes patterns of exercise and daily activities.
■ **Sleep-rest pattern:** Describes patterns of sleep, rest, and relaxation.
■ **Cognitive-perceptual pattern:** Describes patterns of perception and cognition.
■ **Self-perception–self-concept pattern:** Describes self-concept and perception of self-worth, self-competency, body image, and mood state.
■ **Role-relationship pattern:** Describes pattern of role engagements and relationships.
■ **Sexuality-reproductive pattern:** Describes pattern of reproduction and of satisfaction or dissatisfaction with sexuality.
■ **Coping–stress tolerance pattern:** Describes pattern of coping and effectiveness of the pattern in terms of stress tolerance.
■ **Value-belief pattern:** Describes pattern of values, beliefs (including spiritual beliefs), and goals that guide choices and decisions.

The above sequence of patterns provides an order for successful assessment. It begins with the health perception–health management pattern,

including the reason the patient contacted care providers and the understanding of his or her condition. Discussion of self, mood state, relationships, and sexual issues are later in the sequence, when rapport has been
established.

In psychiatric–mental health nursing, the sequence is reversed. Self, mood
state, and relationships are discussed after health perception–health management. These are the topics expected in this setting. Nutrition, elimination, and
activity patterns are important but are assessed later in sequence.

Characteristics of the Health Patterns

- They are easily learned.
- They can be used in all nursing specialties, levels of care, age groups, and
  settings.
- They represent a holistic framework (biopsychosocial-spiritual) of person-
  environment interaction.
- The patterns are influenced by age, culture, gender and, if present, by
  pathophysiology or mental disorder.
- Developmental level and culture are threads found through every pattern
  that shape pattern growth and evolution over the life span.
- The patterns can be used for developmental assessment of an
  individual's, family's, or community's maturation and growth.
- Assessment formats for each disease or clinical area are not needed.
  Using the variables of age, gender, and medical or psychiatric condition,
  the nurse learns which patterns have to be assessed in depth and which
  can be screened with a few questions. For example, cardiac patients
  require in-depth assessment of the activity-exercise pattern.
- Understanding of the health patterns is enriched after experiences across
  age groups, cultures, diseases, and acuity levels.
- They are useful for assessment of individuals, families, and communities.
  Illness can extend to the family and community, and the health of a
  community can affect the individual and family.
- Family and community health patterns are also shaped by developmental
  phases, culture, and the experience of crises or disasters.
- The health patterns are used with nursing theories and data sets required
  by the government; for example, the minimum data set for resident
  assessment and care screening. In addition, the functional health pattern
  assessment complements the database of the biomedical and psychiatric
  assessments.
- The NANDA International Taxonomy II is based on the functional health
  patterns (NANDA, 2007).

Clinical Data, The Nurse, and The Environment

When assessing the health patterns:
- ■ Be clear as to what are good clinical data.
- ■ Remember that you, the nurse, are the sensitive, measuring instrument.
- ■ Consider the environment to ensure privacy and facilitate information sharing.

Clinical Data

Clinical judgments in nursing, medicine, and other health professions are made with less than 100% certainty because of the inherent variability of human behavior. Just collecting more information does not result in certainty. Because of this, nurses:

- ■ Learn to use the most reliable and valid information.
- ■ Know when certain types of information that are cues to health status are needed, such as subjective or objective cues and historical or contextual cues.

Common Cues

- ■ **Reliable cues:** Dependable indicators of a health pattern or diagnosis if obtained through accurate measurement. For example, an accurate recording of food intake at each meal in a hospital situation when no other food is available is a reliable measure of intake. A person's food diary at home may not be reliable.
- ■ **Valid cues:** Represent the property or a characteristic of the pattern being assessed. For example, the patient describes daily food intake. This is a property of the nutritional-metabolic pattern and, therefore, is one valid measure.
- ■ **Subjective cues:** Refer to perceptions, feelings, beliefs, and other reports by the individual, family members, or community representatives.
- ■ **Objective cues:** Refer to care-provider observations, laboratory reports and other tests, and community records.

Nurses value subjective and objective cues for nursing diagnosis; medicine values objective over subjective data for medical diagnosis.

- ■ **Historical cues:** Help to establish a history and are needed to describe a pattern. For example, historical cues establish when pain started, what the blood pressure was in the last year, or a psychotic episode 5 years ago. Avoid historical stereotyping, which is making a judgment on the basis of history alone. Combine historical cues with current state of the patient information.
- ■ **Current state cues:** Help to identify the patient's current state. Current cues combined with historical cues describe a current pattern. Assessing a combination of historical and current cues is useful for predicting risk states.

- **Contextual cues:** Describe situations or significant events, such as a patient's being twice divorced or homeless or a community being a high-crime neighborhood.
- **Diagnostic cues:** Are the critical characteristics of a nursing diagnosis. These cues are few in number. They must be present before making the diagnosis. Diagnostic cues for actual problems are usually current state cues.
- **Supporting cues:** Can increase confidence in the diagnosis. Supporting cues may be a defining characteristic of more than one condition; diagnostic cues are specific to one condition.

When gathering data, remember that quality of information is more important than quantity.

The Nurse

There are a number of characteristics of the nurse that lead to accuracy in assessment. The nurse:

- **Knows what cues to pay attention to during assessment.** The ability to recognize cues to a health condition is based on clinical knowledge. Knowledge of what condition manifests certain signs and symptoms increases sensitivity to those cues and early recognition of the condition.
- **Knows "what predicts what,"** that is, the ability to put information together and predict or anticipate. Knowledge of the likelihood of conditions, events, or relationships is used to predict possible health problems to be investigated during assessment. Age, gender, medical condition, and culture are some of the patient characteristics that allow prediction. To prevent errors, verification follows prediction.
- **Combines** analytic, or logical, reasoning and intuition to interpret assessment data.
- **Verifies** his or her assumptions and intuitive knowing.
- **Organizes** clinical knowledge in his or her memory in a meaningful way for practice. Historically, nurses organized their knowledge into medical categories. Functional health patterns offer a complementary organization of memory stores.
- **Uses** communication and technical skills to ensure accurate assessments and diagnoses. The manner in which questions are asked and the way measurements are taken are important for accuracy of assessment data and the resulting diagnostic judgments.
- **Demonstrates** an empathetic, compassionate manner and establishes a therapeutic relationship. In addition to the humanistic reasons for respect, understanding, and empathy, it is more likely that assessment data will be valid and reliable when there is a good interpersonal interaction with the patient.

- Avoids sharing own similar feelings with the patient, such as by saying, "I have the same problem." This turns the focus to the nurse. The nurse also avoids sharing personal values, politics, or intimacies.

Establishing a Therapeutic Relationship

A therapeutic relationship is a helping relationship wherein the nurse builds trust and rapport by an approach that communicates the following:

- Caring
- Confidence
- Honesty
- Respect
- Confidentiality
- Enthusiasm

With good communication skills, the nurse can develop this kind of relationship with the patient within the first 30 seconds of assessment.

The Environment

To obtain valid information and establish rapport with a new patient, consideration must be given to the environment in which assessment is performed. This applies to the hospital, clinic, home, and community. The following are national guidelines developed by nurses (NICHE Project, 2003, with permission):

Physical Environment

- If possible, ensure that the area in which you are conducting the assessment is at a comfortable temperature and adequately lit with lights that are nonglaring.
- Conduct the assessment in an area free from distractions.
- Ensure proper positioning to maximize the patient's hearing and sight. If necessary, lower the bed to maintain eye-to-eye contact.

Interpersonal Environment

- Ensure proper patient preparation by informing the patient of what will take place and how long it will take.
- Establish comfortable rapport by initiating the evaluation with nonthreatening conversation and presenting yourself in an emotionally nonthreatening manner. This helps to create a patient-professional relationship.
- Watch the pace of assessment, as the rate you ask questions cannot appear hurried. Set the pace by individual patient, if possible.

Timing Considerations

- Timing of assessment should reflect actual cognitive abilities of the individual and not extraneous factors. This may not be possible for an admission assessment in acute or intensive care.
- In order to avoid fatigue, divide assessment if necessary.

- Avoid conducting an assessment during these times:
  - Immediately before or after patient meals.
  - Immediately before or after the patient has had medical, diagnostic, or therapeutic procedures.
  - When the patient is experiencing pain or discomfort.
  - Immediately after a patient awakes from sleep. **After waking a patient, wait 30 minutes before conducting an assessment.**
  - Schedule assessments by appointment when conducting clinic, home, or community-group assessments.

Ethical and Legal Issues in Assessment

In addition to the content, reasoning, and structural aspects of assessment and diagnosis, there are some important ethical and legal issues to be noted.

Ethical Issues

Nurses are morally accountable for their judgments and actions in their practice. This accountability is based on the moral principles of fidelity and respect for dignity, worth, and self-determination. (American Nurses Association, 2002; International Council of Nurses, 2002). Some ethical issues relevant to assessment are:

- **Confidentiality of assessment information:** This is of utmost importance. The passing of the Health Insurance Portability and Accountability Act in 2003 placed this issue in the forefront of health care.
- **Record review:** Patients have the right to review their records at any time. Keep this in mind when documenting assessments and diagnoses. Write only appropriate information. (Although nursing diagnoses are usually done using standardized professional language, nursing diagnoses are usually shared in lay person terminology with the person, family, or community after assessment.)
- **Patient autonomy:** Respect for autonomy and self-determination means that a patient can make an informed decision to refuse to answer an assessment question.

Nurses should not accept delegated functions if they prevent the fulfillment of responsibilities to nursing: assessment, diagnosis, patient care, and documentation.

Legal Issues

Legal aspects of assessment are based on the idea that breach of a duty toward the patient can be viewed as negligence. When negligence results in injury, it can be the basis for legal action. Be aware of some common pitfalls (categories adapted from Eskreis, 1998):

- ■ **Failure to assess:** A tendency exists to assess only the patterns that are directly affected by the medical disease. This is risky. Falls are an example. Assess all patients for the risk of falls, which would normally fall under the health perception–health management pattern, and take precautions.
- ■ **Insufficient monitoring:** Some conditions in problem-focused assessment require frequent monitoring. After an assessment indicating the need for this, write clear orders. In addition, the physician may order specific monitoring; make sure the order is written clearly. Examples of the need for frequent monitoring are suicide risk, self-injury, confusion, and risk for falls.
- ■ **Failure to communicate:** Communication failures can occur in a number of ways, but two situations are most often the cause:
  - ■ **Lack of documentation:** A basic rule to remember is that if a nursing assessment or action was not documented, history will show that the assessment was not performed or no action was taken.
  - ■ **No physician notification:** It is important to communicate significant changes in a patient's physical or mental status to the physician. Signs and symptoms need to be investigated. It is dangerous to assume the physician knows. *Do not assume! Assess and report!*
- ■ **Failure to follow protocols:** Hospitals, localities, and states may have rules for reporting certain behaviors. For example, many states have laws requiring a nurse to immediately report suspicion of patient, child, or elder abuse.

The Nursing History and Examination:
Collection and Interpretation of Information

The nursing history and examination provide a way to organize data collected during the admission assessment. The **nursing history** is obtained through interviewing the patient, family, or community representative. In some cases, the nurse administers a questionnaire or sends the question-naire to the patient's home. The admission interview focuses on areas that require further investigation.

- The **history** is the patient's verbal reports, the subjective data.
- The **examination** provides observations made by the nurse, the objective data.

The nursing history and examination will:

- Organize patient reports and nurse observation into interview and exami-nation, the two sources of information that influence clinical judgment.
- Identify actual or potential problems and strengths.
- Begin to establish a therapeutic relationship.

The Nursing History

Taking a nursing history requires tact and sensitivity. The nurse must put the patient at ease while making sure he or she receives all appropriate informa-tion. Therefore, begin History taking in a friendly, professional manner, and provide smooth transitions across topics. A continual thread throughout the assessment is interpreting the meaning of verbal and nonverbal cues.

Beginning the Nursing History

When preparing to take a nursing history, the nurse must consider:

- **Scope of responsibility as a professional nurse.** This guides the nurse in what to assess. The functional health patterns focus on the nursing domain. The question for assessment is: How is the patient managing his or her health in the 11 areas, and do any problems exist?
- **Manner in which the introduction is made.** The nurse should begin with a greeting that addresses the patient by last name and using Mr., Mrs., or Ms., whichever is appropriate. The nurse should then state his or her name and title in a confident manner.
- **How to best explain purpose.** There are a lot of do's and don't's when explaining the purpose of the nursing history to the patient:

- Do be truthful. For example, say to the patient, "I'd like to talk to you about your health and how you are managing with things like nutrition and daily activities. Could we talk now? Are you comfortable?"
- Do arrange the environment as close to the ideal as possible. (See The Environment in Tab 1.) Insist on privacy for the patient. When scheduling a home visit, arrange for a time when the family member has no distractions.
- Do tell the patient you will be taking notes. Learn to talk and write at the same time to avoid silences during note taking.
- Do not emphasize your task or problems. For instance, do not say:
  - "I have to do an assessment on you."
  - "I need to see if you have any problems."
  - "Before I go off I have to ask you some questions."
- Do not communicate that the history taking will be a "rush job," no matter how many admissions you have.

Smooth Transitions

Try to use smooth transitions from one pattern to another. When using an assessment tool with a checklist, admission interviews can turn into an interrogation, with one question immediately following the previous one. Some ways to begin the interview and to avoid this pitfall are:

- **Begin with a general, open-ended question as a transition from the introduction.** For example, "I know you are [insert reason for admission or home visit], but I was wondering how your general health has been?" Or even more nondirective, "I know this was an emergency admission; how are things now?" Then follow with, "How was your health before?"
- **Write down concerns from this introductory question.** Tell the patient, "Let's write down those things we will want to talk about later." Most concerns can be discussed when the appropriate pattern is assessed.
- **Listen for the patient to elaborate on the current medical problem when asked about his or her health.** This usually occurs during assessment of the health perception–health management pattern. Listen for:
  - How symptoms were managed.
  - How symptoms were interpreted at the time.
  - Understanding of his or her condition.
  - Delay in seeking care.
  - Use of home remedies.

These responses may be areas for health education. Proceed with the next assessment items in the health perception–health management pattern.

- **Use a piece of previously mentioned assessment information for transition.** This technique can allow the nurse to move easily from one pattern to another. For example:

  - Going from the health perception–health management pattern to the nutritional-metabolic pattern: "You mentioned earlier that you wanted to lose weight. Let's go over your typical day's diet. What do you have for breakfast?"
  - Going from the activity-exercise pattern to the sleep-rest pattern: "You keep busy with all those activities. Do you sleep well?"

- **Respond to answers with appropriate clinical advice:** When a patient responds to questions, it is often possible, if time permits, to immediately provide sound clinical advice. For example:

  - A patient reports that he only drinks two glasses of water a day. The nurse responds, "Oh, only two glasses of water a day? You need six to eight; that might be why you are having problems with constipation."
  - A patient complains of incontinence for the last 5 years when getting up, sneezing, or laughing. The nurse responds, "There are some exercises that may help, but first let's have the doctor check that, and then we will talk about the exercises. Do you want to mention that problem to the doctor? Or if you wish, I will tell him to talk to you."

- **Introduce sensitive topics carefully.** The patient will be more comfortable if a sensitive or personal topic is broached with care and concern. The following examples illustrate possible transitions from a role-relationship discussion about family to the sexuality-reproductive pattern:

  - "You mentioned your husband had a cardiac condition. Has this caused any sexual relationship problems?"
  - Less direct: "Have problems in relations with your husband arisen since his illness?"

Questions have to be individualized for the situation. When questions are asked with empathy, both the patient and nurse feel comfortable.

Asking Questions

Different types of questions yield different types of responses. In addition, questions can be designed to elicit different responses during different points in the discussion of a pattern. The same question can elicit a general response at one point and a focused response later in the discussion, when investigating a diagnostic cue.

Open-Ended and Closed-Ended Questions

Open-ended (general) questions are useful at the beginning of a topic when you want the patient to describe something or express concerns. Examples include:

- "How have you been managing since your husband died?"
- "What is it like having a teenager in the house?"
- "Can you tell me more about that?"
- "That must have been difficult." (State this in a caring, questioning manner, and pause for a response.)

In contrast, **closed-ended (focused) questions** elicit a specific response. Examples include:

- "What do you have for breakfast?"
- "When did the pain start?"
- "Are you sleeping well?"

Probing Questions

Probing questions are used with a gentle, empathetic manner. They are necessary to clarify some issue or verify an understanding. This type of question is particularly useful when patients use abstract or medical terms that could have different meanings. Examples include:

- "You mention you are nervous. What do you notice or feel when you are nervous?"
- "What do you experience when you have an ulcer attack?"
- "Many people today worry about sexually transmitted diseases. Do you worry about being at risk?" This question should be asked only when probing is appropriate, indicated by the presence of risk factors.

Confrontational Questions

Confrontational questions should not be used frequently but may be useful when there is a contradiction in the reports. Also, they can be appropriate to bring behavior up for discussion. Examples include:

- "You mentioned before that this started after your divorce 2 years ago. Are you saying it was just a month ago? I must have misunderstood."
- "You sound angry about your work situation. Are you?"
- "I think that was very hard for you. Is that why you made that choice?"

Screening Questions

Screening questions provide a large amount of information about a pattern. They can be used on admission when a full assessment is not possible. For example:

- "Do you feel well rested and ready to go most mornings?" If the patient answers yes, and no other contradictory cues are present, then this is the desired outcome, and no further follow-up questions would be needed.

Clarifying Questions or Observations

Clarifying questions or observations are necessary to prevent misperceptions when patients use vague or ambiguous terms. Otherwise, the nurse might put her or his own meanings and assumptions on the data. For example:

- If a patient responds that he or she is afraid of dying, there are at least four common fears that he or she could be experiencing, all of which require different interventions. Clarification would be necessary, so the nurse would ask: "You know there are a lot of fears around dying. There is pain, who will assume responsibilities, what happens after, and what will happen to my family. Are any of these concerns making you afraid?"
- If a patient responds, "I don't know if it is worth going on," the meaning of this statement is unclear. Avoid responding with a cheery comment, such as: "Of course it is worth going on; you are doing so well." This can close communication. Rather, ask the patient why he or she feels it is not worth going on, and look for signs of depression.

Try to avoid leading questions that reveal the answer you expect. Also be aware of nonverbal communications. For example, nodding of the head can signal that you understand, which can stop the reporting, or it can signal empathy.

Remember that listening is the main feature of a nursing history. Talk only enough to guide the patient in telling his or her health history.

The Examination

Nursing observations during the examination focus on functional health pattern indicators. Repeating the physician's entire physical examination seems inefficient, unless it is being performed for learning purposes. Two important points about indicators are:

- Some are observed during the history, and some require separate attention.
- Others may be indicators of possible problems and explain why certain patterns exist, have changed, or are emerging developmentally.

The examination phase in individual, family, and community assessment verifies or expands the understanding gained during the history. It provides further data, not surprises. The following are a few tips to ensure accuracy:

- Maintain privacy, and drape the patient appropriately. This will help the patient relax.
- Keep a small piece of newsprint in your pocket to test vision.
- In family assessment, examining the home may be important. Ask permission, and try to use something in previous discussion that would be a reason: "You mentioned that you had little space to dress the baby. Could we look at that now?"
- Make sure to use instruments correctly that extend perceptual capabilities, such as the stethoscope.

Interpreting Information

Throughout the nursing history and the examination, the nurse derives meaning from the data to identify problems and plan care. There are various levels of meaning used in analyzing assessment data; all are important because errors can occur at any level: simple evaluation, simple inference, and complex inference are three levels used in analysis.

Simple Evaluation

Simple evaluation determines if a piece of information meets the criterion for health (normal) or not (abnormal). This is done by applying norms, also known as normative criteria. Common norms are:

■ Developmental level.
■ Culture.
■ Gender.
■ Context of the person and situation.

For example: Skin should feel warm and dry. White skin should not have a bluish cast. An individual should brush teeth twice a day. Adults have urinary continence; infants do not.

Simple Inference

Simple inference is a step beyond evaluation. It involves inferential reasoning. For example, consider the following scenario:

■ It is 7:30 a.m. The patient's bed sheets are wrinkled, the blanket is half on the floor, the pillowcase is coming off the pillow, and the patient turns to one side and then the other.

From this scenario the nurse can infer that the patient is restless. Four cues are used to make the inference:

1. Wrinkled bed sheets.
2. Blanket falling on floor.
3. Pillowcase coming off.
4. Patient turning side to side.

Complex Inference

Complex inference involves reasoning and judgment based on clustering multiple cues and inferences. This may result in a nursing diagnosis, either tentative or fully confirmed, or a judgment to be referred to the physician. Consider again the scenario of the restless patient:

■ After determining that the patient was restless, the nurse generated possible explanations, obtained further information from the patient to investigate the possibilities, and then made the following judgment: The patient has Fear (surgical prognosis).

Ending the Admission Assessment

Objectives at the end of the interview and examination are:

■ Give the patient the opportunity to add information by asking if there are any other things he or she would like to mention.
■ Summarize the assessment.
■ Make plans for treatment of the problems identified.

Sharing diagnostic judgments and intervention plans at this time may not be possible. If so, summarize the assessment in a supportive way, using data the patient reported. For example:

■ "Let's both think about what might be causing your family to react this way, and we can talk about it this afternoon."
■ "You've mentioned a number of things; I think you can work out some solutions. Let's talk more about them tomorrow."

In some cases you may be able to say, "You are doing so well! Just keep up the things we talked about, and your blood pressure should be good."

Health Perception–Health Management Pattern

The health perception–health management pattern is similar to an umbrella. Underneath this umbrella are the 10 remaining patterns that are specific to areas of health management.

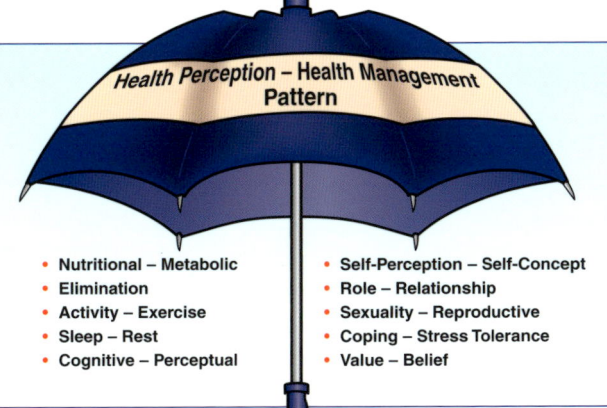

- Nutritional – Metabolic
- Elimination
- Activity – Exercise
- Sleep – Rest
- Cognitive – Perceptual
- Self-Perception – Self-Concept
- Role – Relationship
- Sexuality – Reproductive
- Coping – Stress Tolerance
- Value – Belief

In this pattern the individual, family, or community has an opportunity to identify health-related concerns. This provides the nurse with information on areas that may require in-depth assessment.

Why This Pattern Is Important

The following are reasons that individuals, families, and communities require assessment of this pattern:

- Verifies patient understanding of his or her condition so that misperceptions of illness, treatment, and health-risk management can be clarified.
- Identifies nonadherence to the therapeutic regimen and the reasons.

Some large studies suggest that 50% of people on medication regimens do not adhere to their prescription.

- Identifies need for health teaching.
- Identifies health behaviors and values about health promotion transmitted in the family.
- Identifies community health services and patient access to health education programs, health institutions, and safety programs.

Individual Assessment

The health perception–health management pattern describes the individual's perceived pattern of health and well-being and how health is managed. It includes the individual's perception of his or her health status and its relevance to current activities and future planning. Also included are health-risk management and general health-care behavior, such as:

- Safety practices.
- Adherence to mental and physical health promotion activities.
- Adherence to agreed-upon medical or nursing prescriptions.
- Follow-up care.

Individuals at Risk

Some individuals are at increased risk for problems in this area. Be sensitive to cues when assessing individuals with any of the following characteristics:

- Denial of illness.
- Perceived vulnerability.
- Cognitive impairment.
- Language barrier.
- Visual or hearing deficit.
- Complex therapeutic regimen.
- Elderly, particularly with sensory deficits.
- Lack of knowledge of health policies and resources.
- Nontherapeutic relationship with care provider.

An individualized approach to assessment is necessary. Issues of concern in various cultural, occupational, and age groups can be identified from studies of these groups.

Assessment Items

History

- How has your general health been?
- If appropriate: Most important things done to keep healthy?

- Allergies?
- If person has an illness:
  - Action taken when symptoms perceived? Did that help?
  - What do you think caused this illness?
  - Medications taken currently? Names? Dose? Times?
    - Problems in getting or taking these?
    - Seem to be helping?
    - Did you bring them with you?
- Use herbs or other traditional family remedies?
- Colds in the past year?
- Absences from work or school lasting longer than 1 week?
- Monthly breast self-examination? Prostate screening? Bone density? Colonoscopy?
- If in high-risk group:
  - Flu and pneumonia vaccinations?
  - Tetanus booster?
  - Hepatitis?
  - Other age-appropriate immunizations?
- Use cigarettes? Drugs? Alcohol? When was your last drink?
- Accidents in the past year, either at home, work, or while driving? Wear seat belts?
- Falls in the past year? (See Fall Risk Factor Checklist at the end of this tab to evaluate risk for falls.)
- In the past, easy to find ways to follow doctors' or nurses' suggestions about health management?
- If appropriate: What things are important to you while you are here? How can we be helpful?

Examination
- General appearance.

For in-depth assessment of nonadherence or noncompliance, use the Assessment of Medication and Treatment Self-Management Checklist below.

Diagnostic Categories

The following nursing diagnoses from the NANDA International Taxonomy II (2007) describe diagnostic judgments about individuals. Blue type indicates diagnoses developed by the author, not yet reviewed by NANDA, but found useful in clinical practice (Gordon, 2006).

- **Health-Seeking Behaviors (Specify):** Active seeking (by a person in stable health) of ways to alter personal health habits or the environment to move toward a higher level of health.
- **Risk-Prone Health Behavior:** Inability to modify lifestyle/behaviors in a manner consistent with a change in health status.

■ **Ineffective Health Maintenance (Specify)**: Inability to identify basic health practices, manage own health, or seek help to maintain health.

■ **Ineffective Therapeutic Regimen Management (Specify Area)**: Pattern of regulating and integrating into daily living a program for treatment of illness and its sequelae not meeting specific health goals (specify medication, activity, other treatment regimen, or health promotion disease/prevention).

■ **Risk for Ineffective Therapeutic Regimen Management (Specify Area)**: Presence of risk factors for difficulty in regulating and integrating a treatment or prevention program into daily living.

■ **Readiness for Enhanced Therapeutic Regimen Management**: Pattern of regulating or integrating into daily living a program for treatment of illness and its sequelae that is sufficient for meeting health-related goals and can be strengthened.

■ **Effective Therapeutic Regimen Management (Specify Area)**: Satisfactory pattern of regulating and integrating into daily living a treatment program for illness and its sequelae.

■ **Noncompliance (Specify Area)**: Nonadherence to a therapeutic recommendation following informed decision and expressed intention to attain therapeutic goals (specify drug or treatment program, dietary prescription, observation and reporting of symptoms, follow-up care, health-promoting behaviors).

■ **Risk for Noncompliance (Specify Area)**: Presence of risk factors for nonadherence to therapeutic recommendations following informed decision and expressed intention to adhere or to attain therapeutic goals.

■ **Contamination**: Exposure to environmental contaminants in doses sufficient to cause adverse health effects.

■ **Risk for Contamination**: Accentuated risk for exposure to environmental contaminants in doses sufficient to cause adverse health effects.

■ **Readiness for Enhanced Immunization Status**: Pattern of conforming to local, national, or international standards of immunization to prevent infectious disease(s) that is sufficient to protect a person, family, or community and can be strengthened.

■ **Risk for Infection (Specify Type)**: Presence of increased risk for invasion by pathogenic organisms (specify respiratory, urinary tract, skin).

■ **Risk for Injury**: Presence of risk factors for injury as a result of environmental conditions interacting with adaptive and defensive resources.

■ **Risk for Trauma**: Presence of risk factors for accidental tissue injury, such as a wound, burn, or fracture.

■ **Risk for Falls**: Increased susceptibility for falling that may cause physical harm.

■ **Risk for Perioperative-Positioning Injury**: Presence of risk factors for injury as a result of the environmental conditions found in the perioperative setting.

- ■ **Risk for Poisoning:** Presence of risk factors for accidental exposure to (or ingestion of) drugs or dangerous products in doses sufficient to cause poisoning.
- ■ **Risk for Suffocation:** Presence of risk factors for accidental interruption in the air available for inhalation.
- ■ **Ineffective Protection (Specify):** Decreased ability to guard self from internal or external threats, such as illness or injury.
- ■ **Disturbed Energy Field:** Disruption of the flow of energy surrounding a person's being that results in a disharmony of the body, mind, or spirit.

Family Assessment

Family assessment takes into account all members of the household. It includes their perceptions of:
- ■ Current health and well-being.
- ■ Health risk and disease management.
- ■ Age-appropriate immunizations.
- ■ Health care utilization.

Families at Risk

Some families are at increased risk for problems in this area. Be sensitive to cues when assessing families or groups with any of the following characteristics:
- ■ History of a pattern of absences from school or work.
- ■ Low income.
- ■ No health insurance.
- ■ High housing costs or crowding.

Assessment Items

History
- ■ Family's general health in last few years?
- ■ Family members' colds in the past year?
- ■ Absences from work or school?
- ■ Most important things family does to keep healthy? Do these make a difference to health? (Include family folk remedies.)
- ■ Family members' immunizations? (Check status of adults and children.)
- ■ Regular health-care provider? Frequency of checkups? Adults? Children?
- ■ If children in house: Storage of drugs and cleaning products? Disposal of drugs?

HEALTH
PERCEPT

- Scatter rugs in home? Other home hazards?
- Accidents in the past year, either at home, work, school, or while driving?
- In the past, easy to find ways to carry out doctors' or nurses' suggestions?
- Other things in family's health that are of concern?

Examination

- General appearance of family members.
- Home and yard for safety hazards (with family).
- If appropriate: Medicine storage, cribs, playpens, stove, scatter rugs, and other safety hazards.

For in-depth assessment of home safety, use the Home Environment Safety Checklist below.

Diagnostic Categories

The following nursing diagnosis from the NANDA International Taxonomy II (2007) is used to describe a judgment about the family:

- **Ineffective Family Therapeutic Regimen Management:** Pattern of regulating or integrating into family processes a program for treatment of illness and the sequelae of illness that is unsatisfactory for meeting specific health goals.

Community Assessment

Communities support the health management efforts of individuals and families. Assessment focuses on adequacy of services, such as:

- Health education programs and activities.
- Hospitals, clinics, and other related agencies.
- Public health and future planning.
- School health programs.

Communities at Risk

Some communities are at increased risk for problems in this area. Be sensitive to cues when assessing communities with any of the following characteristics:

- Community budget deficits.
- History of epidemics.
- Heavy industry.

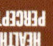

Assessment Items

The following are suggested items for assessing this pattern.

History (Community Representatives)*
- Health and wellness level of the community on a scale of 1 to 5, with 5 being the highest level of health and wellness?
- Major health problems? Particular groups?
- Strong cultural patterns influencing health practices of groups in the area, such as immigrants or the aged with traditional culture?
- People believe they have access to health services?
- Demand for particular health services or prevention programs?
- People believe fire, police, and safety programs sufficient?
- Concerns with air, soil, water, or food contamination?

Examination (Observations and Community Records)
- Morbidity, mortality, longevity, and disability rates (by age groups and sex, if appropriate).
- Accident rates (by district, if appropriate).
- Road conditions.
- Health facilities (by type and age groups, if appropriate).
- Nursing home safety records, including statistics on nurse-resident ratios and falls.
- Hospital infection rates.
- Sanitation codes.
- Food handling, such as at schools, restaurants, and hospitals.
- Public toilet facilities.
- Ongoing health promotion/prevention programs, including utilization rates.
- Ratio of health professionals to population.
- Percentage of people with health insurance.
- Laws regarding drinking age.
- Arrest statistics for drugs, drunk driving.
- Incidence of HIV, AIDS, other sexually transmitted diseases, and tuberculosis.

Diagnostic Categories

The following nursing diagnosis from the NANDA International Taxonomy II (2007) is used to describe judgments about the community:

---

*Community representatives can be residents, families surveyed in their home or in the supermarket, staff of community health-care agencies, and public health department personnel.

- **Ineffective Community Therapeutic Regimen Management (Spec-ify Area):** Pattern of regulating or integrating into community processes programs for treatment of illness and sequelae of illness that are unsatis-factory for meeting health-related goals.

Tips for Assessing This Pattern

- Consider cultural and religious values and beliefs that influence health perception and management.
- Always use assessment data rather than cultural stereotypes in judgments.
- Use open-ended questions to allow the patient to voice his or her concerns.
- Open-ended questions may elicit problems that will be assessed in another pattern. If this occurs, say the concern is important and that you will come back to it. Exceptions to this are emotionally charged concerns that should be talked about when expressed.
- In a nonjudgmental manner, review compliance with medication prescrip-tions: "Let's go over the pills you take. Tell me when you take each one and the dose."
- Use judgment in choosing the time for in-depth assessment of the health management pattern. Determine when the person is ready to think about health promotion. This may or may not be at the admission interview.
- Allow the patient to describe his or her illness and treatment. It is the patient's perception that is needed. Then misperceptions can be corrected.
- In studies of nonadherence, a large percentage of people miss a dose, take less or more than prescribed, or stop taking medications when symptoms are relieved. Try to elicit information about adherence to therapeutic and other nurses' or doctors' recommendations. Recognize that it is difficult for some individuals to admit they did not follow the recommendations. Find out why in a nonjudgmental manner.
- In the hospital, do not use the diagnosis *Noncompliance* when the patient is not able or allowed to manage his or her own medications and treat-ment. A history of noncompliance elicited in the assessment is used as one risk factor for Risk for *Noncompliance* or Risk for *Ineffective Therapeu-tic Regimen Management.*
- To assist in selecting interventions, when using the diagnosis Risk for *Infection,* specify respiratory, skin, urinary tract, childbirth, or wound infection.

In-Depth Assessment Tools

Assessment of Medication and Treatment Self-Management Checklist

What things in your life make it hard to always take the medications or do recommended things? Check all that apply to you:

____Directions are confusing
____There are so many pills to take
____Times are inconvenient
____There is a conflict with my religious beliefs
____It is hard to remember to take some of the pills
____My symptoms went away; I do not need them anymore
____It is hard for me to get to the drugstore to refill
____They have not really helped
____Some people say I focus too much on my health
____The medicine upsets my stomach
____Sometimes it is hard to find money for the medicine
____In my culture we do not do this
____It is hard to tell the doctor/nurse about the problem
____It has been hard to learn how to give myself shots
____They do not realize how this interferes with my family routine
____The medicine makes me feel strange
____I'm so busy; it is hard to always remember

Home Environment Safety Checklist

Check all that apply:

____Throw or scatter rugs not anchored
____Slippery floors
____Littered floors
____Rooms dimly lighted
____Dishes from a few meals piled in sink
____Obstructions on stairs, floors, walkways
____Stair rails broken or unsteady
____Highly waxed floors
____Unsteady chairs or chairs with rollers
____Bathtub/shower without antislip equipment
____Bathtub/shower without handgrips
____Use of cracked dishware or glasses
____Use of thin, worn potholders
____Unanchored electric wires
____Frayed electric wires
____Overloaded fuse boxes

____Faulty electrical plugs
____Electric open plugs not covered (young children)
____Medications not stored safely (young children)
____Defective appliances
____No smoke detectors near bedrooms
____No carbon monoxide detector
____Knives stored with blade uncovered
____Guns or ammunition stored in unlocked area
____Old paint stored in home
____Fuel burning heater not vented to outside
____Inadequately stored combustible or corrosive materials (matches, oily rags)
____Unsafe window protection (young children)
____Large icicles hanging from roof
____Walkways not cleared of ice and snow

Adapted from NANDA, International, 2007 (pp. 232–233).

Fall Risk Factor Checklist

Falls are a risk in the hospital and the home. Assessment of risk factors can determine susceptibility. Check all that apply:
____Age 65 or over
____History of falls
____Use of assistive devices (walker, cane)
____Impaired balance
____Impaired mobility
____Neurovascular foot problems
____Fatigue; sleep deprivation
____Urgency (bowels, urinary)
____Visual problems
____Confusion, dementia
____Alcohol use
____Medications producing sedation
____Cluttered environment
____Dimly lighted room
____No antislip material in bath, shower
____Throw rugs
____Weather conditions (ice, snow)
____Unfamiliar rooms

Adapted from NANDA, International, 2007 (pp. 79–80)

Nutritional-Metabolic Pattern

Food provides fuel for the body's metabolic processes. These processes produce energy for cell maintenance, renewal, and specialized functions of cells.

The nutritional-metabolic pattern evolves from infancy to adulthood and can be influenced by many factors:

- Ethnic heritage and family nutritional patterns can have an impact on food likes and dislikes.
- Positive or negative experiences can become associated with certain foods.
- Radio and television shape attitudes toward foods.
- Community resources can influence access to foods and, through regulations, influence the quality of food.

Why This Pattern Is Important

- Deficiencies in this pattern can explain problems in other areas, such as constipation, skin breakdown, and fatigue. For example, a diet lacking sufficient fluid and roughage may lead to elimination problems.
- Fluid intake is important because metabolism occurs in a fluid medium. Thirst is the first sign of the need for fluids. With increasing age, this sign becomes less effective; assessment of fluid intake during periods of hot weather is important to prevent dehydration.
- Nurses commonly encounter patients who are underweight or obese. Patients who are underweight can suffer from severe nutritional deficiencies, and patients who are overweight are prone to hypertension, diabetes, and orthopedic, workplace, self-esteem, and body-image problems.
- Skin is the first line of defense against infection. Identification of patients at risk for pressure ulcers and detection of any break in the skin are important in preventing infection.
- When there is an interference with cell metabolism, which can result from chemotherapy, protein or vitamin deficiency, and dehydration, repeated skin infections or breakdown can occur.
- To protect the consumer, communities establish regulations for food processing, handling, and refrigeration in transport, food stores, and restaurants.
- Safe food handling and preparation in the home are important to prevent infections.

Individual Assessment

Assessment of the individual focuses on the intake and utilization of food and fluid. This includes:

- Typical daily nutrient intake.
- Types of snacks.
- Eating times.
- Quantity of food and fluids consumed.
- Particular food preferences.
- Use of nutrient, vitamin, and mineral supplements.
- Condition of the skin.

Because of the relatively rapid turnover of cells, skin condition provides a good indicator of nutrient supply to the tissues of the body. Special attention should be given to bony prominences when the individual is not ambulating.

Adequacy of fluid intake and major food groups are judged in relation to metabolic need. Height, weight, body mass index, and waist-to-hip ratio are assessed.

Individuals at Risk

Some individuals are at increased risk for problems in this area. Be sensitive to cues when assessing individuals with any of the following characteristics:

- Impaired swallowing.
- Limited food preparation ability.
- Anorexia.
- Financial limitations.
- Dental caries or missing teeth.
- Chemotherapy with nausea.
- Sedentary activity level.
- Dysfunctional eating patterns.
- Knowledge deficit of nutritional requirements.
- Life stress.
- Immobilization or bedrest.
- Vitamin deficiencies.

History
- Typical daily food intake? (See Food Guide Pyramid below for food groups.)
- Supplements? Vitamins? Type and timing of snacks?
- Weight stable? Loss or gain, including amount? Height loss, including amount?
- Appetite?
- Food or eating discomfort? Problems chewing or swallowing?
- Food coming back?
- Diet restrictions? Able to follow restrictions?
- If appropriate: Breastfeeding?
- Typical daily fluid intake?
- Heal well or poorly?
- Skin problems: Lesions, dryness?
- Dry mouth?
- Dental problems? Bleeding gums? Frequency of dentist visits?

Examination
- Body temperature?
- Bony prominences: Skin intact? (If pressure ulcer present, see Pressure Ulcer Staging at the end of this tab.)
- Lesions? Color?
- Skin: Normal? Dry? Moist?
- Bruises?
- Ankle edema or rings unusually tight?
- Oral mucous membranes: Color? Moistness? Lesions?
- Teeth and gums: General appearance? Alignment of teeth? Dentures? Cavities? Missing teeth?
- Actual weight and height?
- Body mass index? See below.
- Waist-to-hip ratio? See below.
- Intravenous or other type of feeding (specify type)?

Food Pyramid

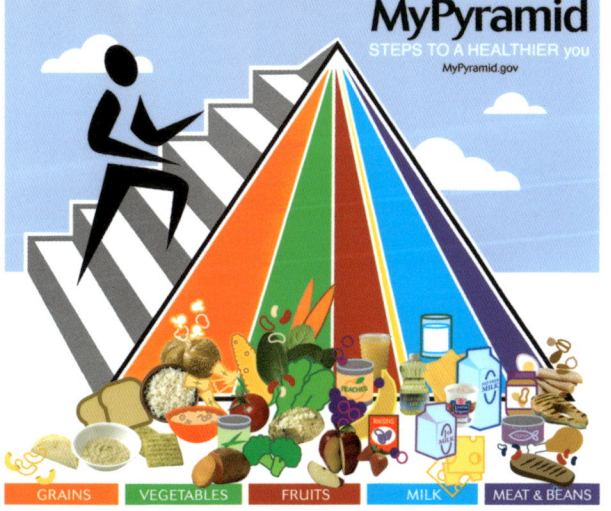

MyPyramid
STEPS TO A HEALTHIER you
MyPyramid.gov

GRAINS | VEGETABLES | FRUITS | MILK | MEAT & BEANS

Diagnostic Categories

The following nursing diagnoses from the NANDA International Taxonomy II (2007) describe diagnostic judgments. Blue type indicates diagnoses developed by the author, not yet reviewed by NANDA, but found useful in clinical practice (Gordon, 2006):

- **Failure to Thrive (Adult):** Progressive functional deterioration of a physical and cognitive nature (associated with multisystem disease that is no longer responsive to medical interventions; condition may respond to psychosocial nursing interventions when diagnosed early).
- **Imbalanced Nutrition: More than Body Requirements or Exogenous Obesity:** Intake of nutrients exceeds metabolic need.

- **Risk for Imbalanced Nutrition: More than Body Requirements or Risk for Obesity:** Presence of risk factors for intake of nutrients that exceeds metabolic need.
- **Imbalanced Nutrition: Less than Body Requirements or Nutritional Deficit (Specify Type):** Insufficient intake of nutrients to meet metabolic need.
- **Readiness for Enhanced Nutrition:** Pattern of nutrient intake that is sufficient for meeting metabolic needs and can be strengthened.
- **Interrupted Breastfeeding:** Break in continuity of breastfeeding process as a result of inability or inadvisability to put baby to breast for feeding.
- **Ineffective Breastfeeding:** Dissatisfaction or difficulty with the breast-feeding process experienced by mother or infant.
- **Effective Breastfeeding:** Mother-infant dyad/family exhibits adequate proficiency and satisfaction with breastfeeding process.
- **Impaired Swallowing (Uncompensated):** Decreased ability to voluntarily pass fluids or solids from the mouth to the stomach.
- **Nausea:** Unpleasant, wavelike sensation in the back of the throat, epigastrium, or throughout the abdomen that may or may not lead to vomiting.
- **Risk for Aspiration:** Risk for entry of gastrointestinal secretions, oropharyngeal secretions, or solids or fluids into tracheobronchial passages.
- **Impaired Oral Mucous Membrane:** Disruption of lips and soft tissue in the oral cavity.
- **Impaired Dentition:** Disruption in tooth development or eruption patterns or structural integrity of individual teeth.
- **Risk for Imbalanced Fluid Volume:** Risk for decrease, increase, or rapid shift among intravascular, interstitial, or intracellular fluid compartments.
- **Excess Fluid Volume:** Increased isotonic fluid retention.
- **Deficient Fluid Volume:** Decreased intravascular, interstitial, or intracellular fluid below normal range for individual (this refers to dehydration–water loss alone without a change in sodium).
- **Risk for Deficient Fluid Volume:** Presence of risk factors for decrease in body fluid (vascular, cellular, or intracellular dehydration).
- **Readiness for Enhanced Fluid Balance:** Pattern of equilibrium between fluid volume and chemical composition of body fluids that is sufficient for meeting physical needs and can be strengthened.
- **Impaired Skin Integrity:** Break in dermis or epidermis.
- **Risk for Impaired Skin Integrity or Risk for Skin Breakdown:** Presence of risk factors for skin ulceration or excoriation.
- **Impaired Tissue Integrity (Specify Type):** Damage to mucous membrane or to corneal, integumentary, or subcutaneous tissue (specify type of tissue and impairment).
- **Pressure Ulcer (Specify Stage):** Break in skin integrity, usually over bony prominences, associated with lying or sitting for prolonged periods.

NUTRI/
METABOLIC

- **Latex Allergy Response:** Allergic response to natural latex rubber products.
- **Risk for Latex Allergy Response:** Risk for allergic response to natural latex rubber products.
- **Ineffective Thermoregulation:** Temperature fluctuation between hypothermia and hyperthermia.
- **Hyperthermia:** Body temperature elevated above normal range.
- **Hypothermia:** Body temperature reduced below normal range.
- **Risk for Imbalanced Body Temperature:** Presence of risk factors for failure to maintain body temperature within normal range.
- **Risk for Impaired Liver Function:** Risk for liver dysfunction.
- **Risk for Unstable Blood Glucose:** Risk for variation of blood glucose/ sugar levels from the normal range.

Family Assessment

Cultural patterns of food selection and preparation are learned early in life within the family. Many times, in order to treat an individual, the family patterns have to be assessed. Assessment focuses on:

- Family pattern of food and fluid intake.
- Mealtime discussions.
- Mealtimes and the presence of family or household members.
- Dietary restrictions and related problems.
- Use of aids, such as meal-delivery services.
- Need for food stamps (if appropriate to situation).

Families at Risk

Some families are at increased risk for dysfunctional or potentially dysfunctional patterns. For example, be sensitive to cues when assessing families with any of the following characteristics:

- Low income.
- Deficient knowledge of daily nutritional requirements.
- Frequent fast-food meals.

Assessment Items

History

- Typical family meal pattern and food intake?
- Supplements, including vitamins and types of snacks?
- Typical family fluid intake?
- Supplements, including fruit juices, soft drinks, and coffee?

- Family member problem with appetite?
- Frequency of dental care of both adults and children?
- Family member with skin problems? Wounds, cuts, scratches, or healing problems?

Examination

When opportunity available, check the following:

- Food types in pantry?
- Refrigerator contents and temperature?
- Meal preparation practices?
- Contents of meal?

Diagnostic Categories

No family diagnoses have been identified in this pattern.

Community Assessment

Communities can influence access to reasonably priced, healthy foods by:

- Encouraging markets to open in the area.
- Ensuring the sanitation of food markets and restaurants.
- Ensuring adequate food refrigeration in markets and restaurants.

Observation in a supermarket during the busy, late afternoon is always informative regarding what foods are purchased. Communities also can encourage stores to accept food stamps and establish meal-delivery services for the homebound.

Assessment focuses on how adequately the community is:

- Ensuring clean water and food.
- Preventing individual and family nutritional deficiencies through social programs and community education.
- Evaluating the nutritional needs of the population.

Communities at Risk

Some communities are at increased risk for problems related to nutrition. Be sensitive to cues when assessing communities with any of the following characteristics:

- Inadequate financial resources (nutritional programs).
- Lack of regulations (safe food handling, refrigeration).
- Lack of inspection or supervision (food stores, water supply, restaurants, street food).

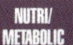

Assessment Items

The following is a guide to community assessment. If data suggest problems, in-depth assessment will be needed. Further assessment is guided by diagnostic possibilities suggested by the assessment data.

History (Community Representatives)
- In general, do most people seem well nourished? Children? Elderly?
- Food supplement programs for low income?
- School nutrition programs?
- Foods reasonably priced in this geographic area, relative to income?
- Dental problems common? Frequency of dental care?
- Stores accessible to most people?
- Meal-delivery services for homebound?
- Water supply and quality? Water-testing services?
- Restaurant food-inspection programs?
- If appropriate: Water usage cost? Drought restrictions? Concern that community growth will exceed good water supply?
- Utility costs manageable for most households? Programs to help?

Examination
- General appearance of people (nutrition, teeth, clothing appropriate to climate)?
  - Children
  - Adults
  - Elderly
- Food purchases (observe check-out counters)?
- Availability of "junk" food machines, including those found within schools?
- Quality of water supply?
- Restaurant inspections?

Diagnostic Categories

No community diagnoses have been identified in this pattern.

Tips for Assessing This Pattern

- Use the food groups in the pyramid to assess intake. Calculations of specific nutrients can be done later if a problem exists.
- Consider that eating is a biopsychosocial-spiritual phenomenon when intake is more or less than body requirements.

- Remember that environmental factors influence a nutritional pattern through culture, religion, and availability of resources in a region. Also, family and community factors can have positive or negative influences on the type of food intake. Assess these.
- Obese patients can encounter bias in health-care settings. Approach assessment of overweight and obese patients with sensitivity.
- Monitor patients who are on bedrest, noting skin condition over bony prominences. If present, stage the status. Constant pressure exceeding capillary pressure will lead to skin breakdown.
- If you discover lesions on the patient during assessment, assess location, time since first noted, size and length, depth, and exudate or signs of infection. Assessment and clear documentation of lesions on admission provide a baseline for measuring the outcome of treatment.

Recognize that complaints of pain or discomfort over a bony prominence when skin is intact can be a sign of deep tissue breakdown.

- Inspect the heels of a person who is not ambulatory (hospital or home). It is difficult to totally remove pressure from the heels when the person moves in bed (Wong & Stotts, 2003).
- Assess malnutrition carefully, particularly in retirement communities and nursing homes. Malnutrition leads to a suppressed immune response and thus to lowered resistance to infection. Studies suggest that many elderly are at risk for malnutrition and dehydration.
- Assess hospitalized patients for nutritional deficits. Patients who are on prolonged fasting for tests or surgery are at particular risk.

In-Depth Assessment Tools

Waist-to-Hip Ratio

The waist-to-hip ratio is used to determine a cardiac risk factor. It is a measurement of waist size divided by hip size.

- Measure the waist at the navel in men and midway between the bottom of the ribs and the top of the hip bone in women.
- Measure hips at the tip of the hip bone in men and at the widest point between the hips and buttocks in women.
- Divide waist size at its smallest by hip size at its largest to obtain the waist-to-hip ratio:
  - Healthy ratio for women is 0.8 or lower; for men 1 or lower.
  - A ratio above 0.85 for women and above 0.90 for men indicates greater risk. Waist circumference greater than 85 cm (35 in) in women and 102 cm (40 in) in men indicates greater than normal risk.

Pressure Ulcer Staging

A pressure ulcer is defined as a localized injury to the skin or underlying tissue, usually over a bony prominence, as a result of pressure or pressure in combination with shear or friction. Pressure ulcers have four stages:

Stage	Description
Stage I	Intact skin with nonblanchable redness of a localized area, usually over a bony prominence. Darkly pigmented skin may not have visible blanching; its color may differ from the surrounding area.
Stage II	Partial-thickness loss of dermis presenting as a shallow, open ulcer with a red-pink wound bed without slough. May also present as an intact or open/ruptured serum-filled blister.
Stage III	Full-thickness tissue loss. Subcutaneous fat may be visible, but bone, tendon, or muscle is not exposed. Slough may be present but does not obscure the depth of tissue loss. May include undermining and tunneling.
Stage IV	Full-thickness tissue loss with exposed bone, tendon, or muscle. Slough or eschar may be present on some parts of the wound bed. Often includes undermining or tunneling.

Note: Ulcers are considered unstageable when the base of the ulcer is covered by slough or eschar (Anderson, Langemo, Hanson, Thompson, and Hunter, 2007).

Body Mass Index (English and Metric)

Body Mass Index (BMI) is an indicator of optimal weight for health. Find the intersection of your weight and height—this is your BMI. Adults with a BMI between 19 and 24 have less risk for illnesses such as heart disease and diabetes than individuals with a BMI between 25 and 29. A BMI greater than 30 indicates greatest risk for obesity-related diseases. Adapted from the National Institute of Health, NHLBI Clinical Guidelines on Overweight and Obesity, June 1988. www.nhlbi.nih.gov/guidelines

Height (feet and inches)

Weight (pounds)	5'0"	5'1"	5'2"	5'3"	5'4"	5'5"	5'6"	5'7"	5'8"	5'9"	5'10"	5'11"	6'0"	Weight (kilograms)
100	20	19	18	18	17	17	16	16	15	15	14	14	14	45
105	21	20	19	19	18	17	17	16	16	16	15	15	14	47
110	21	21	20	19	19	18	18	17	17	16	16	15	15	50
115	22	22	21	20	20	19	19	18	17	17	17	16	16	52
120	23	23	22	21	21	20	19	19	18	18	17	17	16	54
125	24	24	23	22	21	21	20	20	19	18	18	17	17	57
130	25	25	24	23	22	22	21	20	20	19	19	18	18	59
135	26	26	25	24	23	22	22	21	20	19	19	19	18	61
140	27	26	26	25	24	23	23	22	21	20	20	20	19	63
145	28	27	27	26	25	24	23	23	22	21	21	20	20	66
150	29	28	27	27	26	25	24	23	23	22	22	21	20	68
155	30	29	28	27	27	26	25	24	24	23	22	22	21	70
160	31	30	29	28	27	27	26	25	24	24	23	22	22	72
165	32	31	30	29	28	27	27	26	25	24	24	23	22	75
170	33	32	31	30	29	28	27	27	26	25	24	24	23	77
175	34	33	32	31	30	29	28	27	27	26	25	24	24	79
180	35	34	33	32	31	30	29	28	27	27	26	25	24	82
185	36	35	34	33	32	31	30	29	28	27	27	26	25	84
190	37	36	35	34	33	32	31	30	29	28	27	27	26	86
195	38	37	36	35	33	32	31	31	30	29	28	27	26	88
200	39	38	37	35	34	33	32	31	30	30	29	28	27	91
205	40	39	37	36	35	34	33	32	31	30	29	29	28	93
210	41	40	38	37	36	35	34	33	32	31	30	29	28	95
215	42	41	39	38	37	36	35	34	33	32	31	30	29	98
220	43	42	40	39	38	37	36	34	33	32	32	31	30	100
225	44	43	41	40	39	37	36	35	34	33	32	31	31	102
230	45	43	42	41	39	38	37	36	35	34	33	32	31	104
235	46	44	43	42	40	39	38	37	36	35	34	33	32	107
240	47	45	44	43	41	40	39	38	36	35	34	33	33	109
245	48	46	45	43	42	41	40	38	37	36	35	34	33	111
250	49	47	46	44	43	42	40	39	38	37	36	34	34	114
	150	152.5	155	157.5	160	162.5	165	167.5	170	172.5	175	177.5	180	

Height (centimeters)

☐ Underweight ☐ Weight Appropriate ☐ Overweight ☐ Obese

Elimination Pattern

Elimination is a biopsychosocial behavior. Child-rearing books devote many pages to the subject, and children learn social rules:

- Where elimination should take place.
- Socially defined structures to be used.
- Care of the body following elimination.
- Respect for privacy.
- When proper and not proper to discuss the subject.
- Psychologically, privacy and control of elimination become important. Recognize this when assessing an adult who experiences incontinence. The focus for assessment of individuals, families, and communities is on excretion and waste disposal.

Why This Pattern Is Important

The following are reasons that individuals, families, and communities require assessment of this pattern:

- Intake and output measurements provide information on fluid balance and may signal fluid retention.
- Anxiety, depression, and social isolation can result from urinary and fecal incontinence. Loss of control is frequently referred to as the "unvoiced symptom."
- *Nearly one-third of adult women older than 65 years experience some urinary incontinence. Men experience less. Ratio of the problem in females to males younger than 60 years is about 4:1. In those 60 years and older, the ratio is 2:1. Fecal incontinence has a prevalence of about 10% in adults. Nearly half of adults living in nursing homes have problems in control of either bladder or bowel.
- Urinary or fecal incontinence can produce skin irritation, which leads to breakdown and ulceration.
- Retention of urine can occur with lower abdominal or pelvic surgery.
- Infection can spread through a family if there is inadequate disposal of wastes.
- Inadequate disposal of wastes in industry can pollute the air or contaminate ground water.

Individual Assessment

Elimination is the way the body controls fluid and chemical composition and the excretion of the products of metabolism. Assessment focuses on:

*Wyman et al, 2004.

- Bowel, bladder, and skin excretion.
- Regularity of urination and bowel evacuation.
- Color, quality, and quantity of urine and feces.
- Aids used to facilitate function, such as routines, devices, and methods to control excretion.
- Changes or disturbances in bowel or bladder elimination.

Individuals at Risk

Some individuals are at risk for elimination problems. Be sensitive to cues when assessing individuals with any of the following characteristics:

- Elderly with neuromuscular changes in pelvic floor muscles.
- Spinal cord injury.
- Impaired mobility.
- Cognitive impairment.
- Diabetes mellitus with neurological changes.
- Multiple sclerosis.
- Prostatectomy.
- Prostate enlargement.
- Lower abdominal and pelvic surgery.
- Female who has had multiple births.
- Radiation cystitis.

Assessment Items

History
- Bowel elimination pattern: Frequency? Character? Discomfort?
- Problem in control?
- Lose bowel contents when unwanted? (Describe bowel continence using Classification of Bowel or Bladder Continence at the end of this tab.)
- Use of laxatives? Other methods to maintain regularity?
- Urinary elimination pattern? (Describe bladder continence using Classification of Bowel or Bladder Continence at the end of this tab.) Frequency?
- Trouble holding urine until getting to bathroom?
- Lose urine when unwanted, such after sneezing, coughing, or laughing? If yes: Wear a pad?
- Excess perspiration? Odor problems?
- Body cavity drainage from catheter, ostomy, or suction?

Examination
- If indicated: Examine excreta or drainage as to its color, amount, and consistency.

Diagnostic Categories

The following nursing diagnoses from the NANDA International Taxonomy II (2007) describe diagnostic judgments. Blue type indicates diagnoses developed by the author, not yet reviewed by NANDA, but found useful in clinical practice (Gordon, 2006).

- **Constipation:** Decrease in frequency of defecation accompanied by difficult or incomplete passage of hard, dry stool.
- **Perceived Constipation:** Self-diagnosis of constipation and ensures daily bowel movement through abuse of laxatives, enemas, or suppositories.
- **Intermittent Constipation Pattern:** Periodic episodes of hard, dry stools not associated with a pathological state.
- **Risk for Constipation:** Presence of risk factors for a decrease in frequency of defecation and difficult or incomplete passage of stool or passage of excessively hard, dry stool.
- **Diarrhea:** Passage of loose, unformed stools.
- **Bowel Incontinence:** Change in bowel habits characterized by involuntary passage of stool.
- **Impaired Urinary Elimination:** Involuntary loss of urine at somewhat predictable intervals when a specific bladder volume is reached.
- **Functional Incontinence:** Inability of usually continent person to reach toilet in time to avoid unintentional loss of urine.
- **Reflex Incontinence:** Involuntary loss of urine at somewhat predictable intervals when a specific bladder volume is reached.
- **Overflow Urinary Incontinence:** Involuntary loss of urine associated with overdistention of the bladder.
- **Stress Incontinence:** Involuntary loss of urine of less than 50 mL occurring with increased abdominal pressure.
- **Urge Incontinence:** Involuntary passage of urine occurring soon after a strong sense of urgency to void.
- **Risk for Urge Incontinence:** Risk for involuntary loss of urine associated with a sudden, strong sensation of urgency.
- **Total Urinary Incontinence:** Continuous and unpredictable loss of urine.
- **Urinary Retention:** Incomplete emptying of the bladder.
- **Readiness for Enhanced Urinary Elimination:** Pattern of urinary functions that is sufficient for meeting eliminatory needs and can be strengthened.

Family Assessment

The elimination pattern of a family involves handling of wastes and disposal of hazardous and nonhazardous materials, which has to be done in a way that does not risk infection and contaminate the environment. The focus of assessment is on:

- Family disposal of garbage.
- Disposal of human and animal waste, including kitchen and bathroom waste disposal and related hygienic practices.
- Family avoidance of disposal practices that would contribute to environmental pollution, such as oil paint and computer ink cartridges.

Families at Risk

Some families are at increased risk for problems in this area. Be sensitive to cues when assessing families with any of the following characteristics:

- Lack of toilet hygiene.
- Improper animal waste disposal.
- Inadequate water temperature when washing dishes and clothes.
- Open garbage that attracts flies.

Assessment Items

History
- Problems in waste and garbage disposal?
- Adequate disposal of pet waste, both indoor and outdoor?
- Problems with flies, roaches, rodents, or indoor air pollution?
- Able to get adequately hot water for washing dishes and clothes?

Examination
- Toilet facilities?
- Garbage disposal?
- Pet waste disposal?
- Indicators of risk for flies, roaches, rodents?

Diagnostic Categories

No family diagnoses have been identified in this pattern.

Community Assessment

In most countries of the world, there is heightened sensitivity to pollution of the air, soil, and water. Assessment of the community elimination pattern focuses on community programs in the following areas:

- Community industrial and other wastes that can be carried in the atmosphere to other communities.

- Auto emissions that can pollute the air and be a risk for people with respiratory problems.
- Inadequate waste disposal that can contaminate groundwater.
- Workers who can be exposed to chemicals or airborne dusts if safety precautions are not taken.

Communities at Risk

Some communities are at increased risk for problems in this area. Be sensitive to cues when assessing communities with any of the following characteristics:

- Underdeveloped sanitation codes.
- Absence of laws protecting food, water supply, and the environment.
- History of industrial air, water, and ground contamination.

Assessment Items

History (Community Representatives)
- Major kinds of wastes, such as industrial waste and sewage?
- Disposal systems?
- Recycling programs?
- Problems perceived by community?
- Pest control?
- Food service inspection, such as inspection of restaurants and street vendors?

Examination (Community Records)
- Communicable-disease statistics.
- Air pollution statistics.

Diagnostic Categories

The following nursing diagnoses from the NANDA International Taxonomy II (2007) are classified under health management as they focus on adverse health effects experienced by the individual. See related factors and risk factors for environmental contamination.

- **Contamination:** Exposure to environmental contaminants in doses sufficient to cause adverse health effects.
- **Risk for Contamination:** Accentuated risk for exposure to environmental contaminants in doses sufficient to cause adverse health effects.

Tips for Assessing This Pattern

- Think about food and fluid intake (nutritional-metabolic pattern) and activity (activity-exercise pattern) when investigating an elimination problem. Constipation can be caused by lack of activity and food and fluid intake.
- Dehydration can result from too little intake for metabolic need.
- The type of urinary incontinence has to be identified to select the correct interventions. Types of incontinence are functional, reflex, stress, urge, and overflow. See Comparison Table for differential diagnosis of incontinence below.
- Stress and urge incontinence interfere with life activities. Because people are embarrassed to talk about incontinence or think no help is available, it is underdiagnosed and underreported by care providers. Do a full assessment. See Comparison Table for Differential Diagnosis of Incontinence below.
- Urinary tract infection is common in women. Be alert for symptoms, such as pain and burning upon urination, frequency, and blood in the urine. Investigate possible reasons as a basis for referral to physician and patient health education.
- Onset of confusion in an elderly patient may signal a urinary tract infection.
- Distinguish between the current presence of constipation and the report of episodes of constipation. Use the diagnosis *Constipation* to describe the former and *Intermittent Constipation* for the latter.

In-Depth Assessment Tools

Classification of Bowel or Bladder Continence

Grade	Classification	Description
0	Continent	Complete control of bladder and bowel. Does not use any type of catheter or other urinary collection device.
1	Continent with device or bladder program	Complete control with use of catheter, urinary collection device, ostomy, or toileting program.
2	Usually continent	Bladder incontinence episodes once a week or less. Bowel incontinence less than weekly.
3	Occasionally incontinent	Bladder incontinence two or more times a week but not daily. Bowel incontinence once a week.
4	Incontinent	Unable to control bladder or bowel.

Comparison Table for Differential Diagnosis of Incontinence	
Type of Incontinence	**Description**
Functional incontinence	When need to void, unable to get to toilet quickly. Cognitive impairment sometimes present.
Reflex incontinence	Specific to spinal cord injury above 3rd sacral. Unaware of bladder fullness; spinal reflex (without higher-level control).
Stress incontinence	Sudden loss with increased abdominal pressure due to exertion, laughing, coughing. Also may be dribbling with loss of small amounts.
Urge incontinence	Sudden overwhelming urge to urinate. Cannot control voiding long enough to reach toilet. Urine leakage en route to toilet.
Overflow incontinence	Bladder overfills and leakage of small amounts. Bladder distention on examination.
Total incontinence	Unaware of urge to void. Continuous, involuntary loss.
Mixed incontinence	May have combination of urge and stress urinary incontinence.

Activity-Exercise Pattern

The activity-exercise pattern describes three functions that are important to everyone's daily life:

- **Mobility:** Brings independence. When challenged by illness, can affect nearly all other health patterns.
- **Independent self-care:** One of the major activities of daily living.
- **Exercise and leisure:** Bring diversion and social interaction.

Underlying all activities is the important concept of *energy expenditure,* which requires four main support systems:

- Neurological system.
- Musculoskeletal system.
- Cardiovascular system.
- Respiratory system.

For families, the activity-exercise pattern involves sharing and managing:

- Daily routines.
- Shopping.
- Cooking.
- Meal planning.
- Cleaning.
- Home management.
- Leisure activities.

Communities also have a sense of activity and movement. This can be hectic, as in the traffic patterns of city life, or pastoral, as in country life. Also, communities support the activity-exercise patterns of individuals and families by providing:

- Parks and recreational facilities.
- Access to shopping.
- Means of transportation.
- Low-cost housing.

Why This Pattern Is Important

The following are reasons that individuals, families, and communities require assessment of this health pattern:

- It is estimated that about one-fifth of the population has some disability involving mobility or self-care. Assessment of risk factors and prevention of disabilities have to begin in early adulthood in order to prevent problems in later life.
- Assessment can reveal lack of sufficient exercise, which leads to:
  - Poor muscle tone.

ACTIVITY/
EXERCISE

- Problems in balance.
- Feelings of mental and physical fatigue.
- Minimal exercise, sedentary work or school activities, and an imbalanced nutritional pattern can lead to obesity. These are major risk factors for coronary artery disease or cerebrovascular accident. Decreased activity tolerance and impaired mobility can result.
- Assessment of work skills and extent of disability is the basis for vocational rehabilitation counseling.
- Older adults with poor balance and poor muscle tone in the legs and hips are at risk for falls.
- Foot problems are common, particularly in females. Assessment of the feet and ankle joints is required because foot problems impair:
  - Balance.
  - Mobility.
  - Activity and exercise tolerance.
- Foot problems, such as painful corns, calluses, and toe deformities, decrease activity tolerance and impair mobility. Referral to a podiatrist may be indicated.
- Assessment of range of joint motion identifies the risk for contractures (shortening of tendons at movable joints).
- Lack of community transportation can limit access to health-care services.
- For the disabled, facilitation of independent self-care and locomotion rests on accurate assessment of family caregiver knowledge and the home and neighborhood environment.
- The extent to which community and government programs meet the needs of the disabled requires continual assessment and advocacy.

The activity-exercise pattern describes an individual's activity tolerance and daily exercise pattern. The following specific self-care abilities are assessed:

- Feeding.
- Bathing-hygiene.
- Dressing-grooming.
- Toileting.

Also included are:

- Home management.
- Shopping.
- Type, quantity, and quality of exercise.
- Leisure activities.
- Complex functions of four supporting systems: cardiac, pulmonary, musculoskeletal, and neurological.

Some individuals are at increased risk for problems in this pattern. Be sensitive to cues when assessing individuals with any of the following characteristics:

- Imbalance between cellular oxygen supply and demand, such as from cardiovascular or pulmonary conditions.
- Long-term bedrest or wheelchair usage or deconditioning due to sedentary lifestyle.
- Leg cramps with ambulation, indicative of circulatory problems.
- Decreased sensation to extremities, such as from diabetic neuropathy.
- Uncompensated paralysis and weakness, such as from cerebrovascular accident, spinal cord injury, or brain tumor.
- Cognitive deficit, such as wandering with dementia.
- Uncompensated musculoskeletal condition, such as fractures.
- Confusion, coma.
- Environmental barriers to self-care or mobility.
- Situational depression.
- Conditions resulting in loss of eyesight.
- High job or family demands leaving "no time for exercise."

History
- Sufficient energy for desired and required activities around work, school, and home?
- Describe activity level for most days of the week:
  - Very active.
  - Moderately active.
  - Mostly sedentary.
- Exercise pattern? Type? Regularity? Hours per week?
- Leisure activities: Type? Alone or with others?
- In last few months: Unsteady gait? Dizziness? Fainting? Falls?
- Patient's perceived ability for (code 1 to 4 according to Functional Levels Code below):
  - Feeding____
  - Bathing____
  - Toileting____
  - Bed mobility____
  - Dressing____
  - Grooming____
  - General mobility____
  - Cooking____
  - Home maintenance____
  - Shopping____

Functional Levels Code	
Grade	**Description**
0	Independent
1	Requires use of equipment or device
2	Requires assistance or supervision of another person
3	Requires assistance or supervision of another person and equipment or device
4	Is dependent and does not participate

From Gordon 2006, p, 174. Formerly NANDA International, 2005.

Examination*

- Pulse: Rate, rhythm, and strength.
- Blood pressure.
- Respiration: Rate, rhythm, depth.
- Breath sounds.
- Hand-grip strength.
- Small-muscle dexterity: Can pick up pencil.
- Muscle firmness (tone).
- Range of motion (joints): No impairment, localized (specify location), impaired on one side, or impaired on both sides.
- Motor-function: No impairment, localized (specify location), impaired on one side, or impaired on both sides.
- Absent body part, such as extremities, fingers, or toes.
- Gait.
- Posture
- Mobility:
  - Bedrest: Unable to move independently.
  - Bed mobility: While in bed, can turn side to side and position body.
  - Ambulatory.
  - Ambulatory with cane, walker, or crutches.
  - Wheelchair.

Diagnostic Categories

The following nursing diagnoses from the NANDA International Taxonomy II (2007) describe diagnostic judgments. Blue type indicates diagnoses developed by the author, not yet reviewed by NANDA, but found useful in clinical practice (Gordon, 2006):

*Some assessment items are adapted from Morris (1990).

- **Activity Intolerance (Specify Level):** Abnormal response to energy-consuming body movements involved in required or desired daily activities.
- **Risk for Activity Intolerance:** Presence of risk factors for abnormal response to energy-consuming body movements.
- **Fatigue:** Overwhelming sustained sense of exhaustion and decreased capacity for physical and mental work at usual level.
- **Sedentary Lifestyle:** Reports a habit of life that is characterized by a low physical activity level.
- **Deficient Diversional Activity:** Decreased engagement in recreational or leisure activities.
- **Impaired Physical Mobility (Specify Level):** Limitation of independent, purposeful body movement in the environment.
- **Impaired Walking (Specify Level):** Limitation of independent movement within the environment on foot or with a device such as a cane, crutches, or walker.
- **Impaired Wheelchair Mobility:** Impairment of independent operation of wheelchair within the environment.
- **Impaired Bed Mobility (Specify Level):** Limitation of independent movement from one bed position to another.
- **Impaired Transfer Ability (Specify Level):** Limitation of independent body movement between two nearby surfaces.
- **Wandering:** Meandering, aimless, or repetitive locomotion that exposes the individual to harm; frequently incongruent with boundaries, limits, or obstacles and may be sporadic or continued.
- **Risk for Disuse Syndrome:** Presence of risk factors for deterioration of body systems as the result of prescribed or unavoidable musculoskeletal inactivity.
- **Risk for Joint Contractures:** Presence of risk factors for shortening of tendons at movable joints (back, head, upper and lower extremities).
- **Total Self-Care Deficit (Specify Level):** Inability to complete feeding, bathing, toileting, dressing, and grooming of self.
- **Bathing-Hygiene Self-Care Deficit (Specify Level):** Impaired ability to perform or complete bathing and hygiene activities.
- **Dressing-Grooming Self-Care Deficit (Specify Level):** Impaired ability to perform or complete dressing and grooming activities.
- **Feeding Self-Care Deficit (Specify Level):** Impaired ability to perform or complete feeding activities.
- **Toileting Self-Care Deficit (Specify Level):** Impaired ability to perform or complete toileting activities.
- **Readiness for Enhanced Self-Care:** Pattern of performing activities for oneself that helps to meet health-related goals and can be strengthened.
- **Delayed Surgical Recovery:** Extension of the number of postoperative days required for individuals to initiate and perform activities that maintain life, health, and well-being.

- ■ **Impaired Home Maintenance:** Inability to maintain a safe, growth-promoting immediate environment (specify mild, moderate, severe, risk, or chronic).
- ■ **Dysfunctional Ventilatory Weaning Response (DVWR):** Inability to adjust to lower levels of mechanical ventilator support, which interrupts and prolongs the weaning process (specify mild, moderate, severe).
- ■ **Impaired Spontaneous Ventilation:** Decreased energy reserves result in an individual's inability to maintain breathing adequate to support life.
- ■ **Ineffective Airway Clearance:** Inability to effectively clear secretions or obstruction from respiratory tract.
- ■ **Ineffective Breathing Pattern:** Inspiration or expiration that does not provide adequate ventilation.
- ■ **Impaired Gas Exchange:** Excess or deficit in oxygenation or carbon dioxide elimination at the alveolar-capillary level.
- ■ **Decreased Cardiac Output:** Inadequate blood pumped by the heart to meet the metabolic needs of the body.
- ■ **Ineffective Tissue Perfusion (Specify Type):** Decrease in blood supply at the capillary level resulting in failure to nourish tissues.
- ■ **Autonomic Dysreflexia:** Life-threatening, uninhibited, sympathetic nervous system response to a noxious stimulus with a spinal cord injury of T7 or above.
- ■ **Risk for Autonomic Dysreflexia:** Risk for life-threatening, uninhibited, sympathetic nervous system response to a noxious stimulus with a spinal cord injury of T7 or above (following spinal shock; has been demonstrated with injuries at T7 or above).
- ■ **Risk for Peripheral Neurovascular Dysfunction:** Presence of risk factors for disruption in circulation, sensation, or motion of an extremity, such as a cast or bandage being too tight.
- ■ **Decreased Intracranial Adaptive Capacity:** Repeated disproportionate increases in intracranial pressure in response to noxious and non-noxious stimuli due to lack of compensation for increases in intracranial volumes by intracranial fluid dynamic mechanisms.

Family Assessment

The activity-exercise pattern describes family pattern of activity, exercise, leisure, and recreation. It includes how the family budgets time and resources in order to organize its activities of daily living, such as:

- ■ Working.
- ■ Dependent care.
- ■ Self-care.
- ■ Cooking.
- ■ Shopping.
- ■ Cleaning.
- ■ Home maintenance.

The emphasis of assessment is on activities of major importance or significance and the presence of any limitations.

Families at Risk

Some families are at increased risk for problems in this area. Be sensitive to cues when assessing families or groups with any of the following characteristics:

- Time constraints, such as two jobs.
- Knowledge deficit (time management).
- Fatigue.
- Member with disability.
- Insufficient budgeting of family finances.

Assessment Items

History
- Problems in:
  - Shopping, including transportation to and from store?
  - Schedule keeping for members, such as for children's activities?
  - Cooking and meal preparation?
  - Keeping up the house?
  - Budgeting income for food, clothes, home, and other costs?
- Approximately how many hours per week do family members find time to exercise? Type? Regularity?
- Family leisure activities? Active activities, such as sports and walking, or passive activities, such as television and computer games?
- If relevant: Any difficulty managing care-taking activities of children or other dependent family members, such as those with a disability?

Examination
- General appearance of home maintenance?
- Personal maintenance of members who are present?

Diagnostic Categories*

No family diagnoses have been identified in this pattern. Two diagnoses may be relevant for families in the child-rearing phase:

- **Developmental Delay in Self-Care Skills**: Demonstrates deviations from age-group norms for self-care skills.
- **Risk for Sudden Infant Death Syndrome:** Presence of risk factors for sudden death of an infant.

---

*NANDA International, 2007; Gordon, 2006.

ACTIVITY/
EXERCISE

Community Assessment

The activity-exercise pattern describes the type, quantity, and quality of leisure and recreation programs available to various age groups in the community. These include senior centers and teenage recreation programs. Included also are housing and transportation that support mobility for various income levels and the disabled.

Communities at Risk

Some communities are at increased risk for problems in this area. Be sensitive to cues when assessing communities with any of the following characteristics:

- High crime rates that restrict mobility.
- High rates of juvenile delinquency.
- Low-budget rehabilitative services.
- Inadequate transportation services.

Assessment Items

History (Community Representatives)
- Is transportation convenient and affordable for:
  - Work?
  - Shopping?
  - Recreation?
  - Health care?
- People use community centers and playgrounds?
  - Seniors?
  - Children?
  - Adults?
- Is housing adequate? Available? Cost?
- Low-income housing? Senior housing?

Examination
- Recreation and cultural programs?
- Availability of nursing homes?
- Assistive living facilities?
- Senior center with exercise and recreational programs?
- Affordable housing?
- Curbs and bathrooms that are wheelchair-accessible?
- Traffic lights that play a sound when changing to facilitate the blind who are learning mobility?

- Elevators in community buildings that enable persons with activity intolerance to visit for business or recreation?
- Child-care resources available?
- Rehabilitation facilities relative to population needs?
- External maintenance of streets, homes, yards, and apartment houses?
- Transportation services relative to need?

Diagnostic Categories

No community diagnoses have been identified in this pattern.

Tips for Assessing This Pattern

- Use the Functional Levels Code (see Individual Assessment above) when assessing self-care abilities and other activities of daily living. Use the same coding system for stating outcomes and for evaluating outcome attainment.
- Assessment reveals the usual sequence of returned function after a stroke to be:
  - Feeding.
  - Continence.
  - Toileting.
  - Bathing.
  - Dressing.
  - Cooking.
  - Shopping.
  - Home maintenance.

The above is from lesser to greater complexity. The more complex functions return later (McCourt, 1993).

- Code impaired mobility on admission using the Functional Levels Code. Use the same coding system for stating outcomes and for evaluating outcome attainment.
- Cardiac and pulmonary medical conditions produce self-care deficits. A clinically useful way of describing this problem is *Self-care deficit* (Level 2) *related to activity intolerance.* The patient learns to compensate through energy conservation.
- Cerebrovascular accident may result in self-care deficits and impaired mobility. A clinically useful way of describing this problem for nursing and physical therapy is *Self-care deficit* (Level 3) *related to uncompensated hemiplegia.* The patient learns to compensate through rehabilitation.
- Assess in greater depth when identifying these conditions:

ACTIVITY/
EXERCISE

- Impaired gas exchange.
- Decreased cardiac output.
- Ineffective tissue perfusion.
- Decreased intracranial adaptive capacity.

For example, with decreased cardiac output, nursing assessment may reveal one or more of the following:

- Activity intolerance.
- Self-care deficit.
- Knowledge deficit.
- Anxiety, fear, or death anxiety.
- Ineffective management of therapeutic regimen.
- Disturbed self-esteem or body image.
- When unhealthy conditions are found on a home visit, assessment of family home maintenance requires sensitivity. Identifying reasons for the situation may be the best assessment approach rather than critiquing the conditions themselves.

In-Depth Assessment Tools

Borg Scale for Rating Perceived Shortness of Breath

Directions: This tool is useful for evaluating a patient who complains of shortness of breath on exertion. Instruct the patient to look at the scale and rate his or her dyspnea (6 and 8 are amounts of severity).

Grade	Description
0	Nothing
0.5	Very, very slight (just noticeable)
1	Very slight
2	Slight
3	Moderate
4	Somewhat severe
5	Severe
6	
7	Very severe
8	
9	Very, very severe
10	Very, very severe (almost maximum)

From Borg GA (1982). Borg Scale. Med Sci Sports Exerc 14:377–387, with permission.

Grading Dyspnea

Directions: Use the following table to help the patient describe how various activities, weather patterns, or other factors affect his or her breathing. Keeping a diary between clinic or office visits may be helpful to identify needs for learning energy-conservation methods.

Grade	Indications
0	Not troubled by breathlessness except with strenuous exercise.
1	Troubled by shortness of breath when hurrying on a level path or walking up a slight hill.
2	Walks more slowly on a level path because of breathlessness than do people of the same age or has to stop to breathe when walking on a level path at own pace.
3	Stops to breathe after walking about 100 yards on a level path.
4	Too breathless to leave the house or breathless when dressing or undressing.

Functional Capacity Assessment of Activity Tolerance

Directions: This classification is widely used in cardiac care and is useful for nurses when assessing activity intolerance. It is also useful for before-and-after measures when recommending conditioning exercises or progression in a cardiac rehabilitation program.

Class	Limitation	Indications
1	No limitation	Ordinary physical activity does not cause undue fatigue, palpitation, dyspnea, or anginal pain.
2	Slight limitation	Comfortable at rest. Ordinary physical activity results in fatigue, palpitation, dyspnea, or anginal pain.
3	Marked limitation	Comfortable at rest. Less than ordinary activity causes fatigue, palpitation, dyspnea, or anginal pain.
4	Severe limitation	Inability to carry on any physical activity without discomfort. May have symptoms of heart failure or anginal syndrome at rest.

ACTIVITY/
EXERCISE

Sleep-Rest Pattern

Sleep is restorative. Theories from sleep research suggest that during sleep:

■ The body repairs and renews cells.
■ New information from short-term memory is organized and integrated into long-term memory by the brain (Hodgson, 1991).

Usually, adults require 7 to 8 hours of sleep per day. Specific amounts vary with lifestyle and health condition. The focus of the sleep-rest pattern assessment is on whether the person feels rested and ready for the day's activities.

Why This Pattern Is Important

■ Fast-paced societies are associated with higher percentages of people with sleep deprivation. Some busy people see sleeping as a waste of time. A small percentage of people may need referral to a specialist for sleep disturbances, such as sleep apnea.
■ Changes in sleep patterns occur with admission to hospitals and other health-care facilities. Hospitalized patients can experience frequent sleep interruptions that lead to sleep deprivation.
■ The benefit of the afternoon nap as a response to postprandial (after meals) lethargy is being recognized by some businesses, which are making allowances for power naps of 20 minutes.
■ Pain, anxiety, and fear are common causes of sleep deprivation.
■ Communities can require regulations that decrease the amount of noise near residential neighborhoods.
■ Overcrowded sleeping arrangements or noise in a home can lead to sleep deprivation.

Individual Assessment

The sleep-rest pattern describes:

■ Quality of sleep time.
■ Quantity of sleep.
■ Rest and relaxation or quiet periods during the day.
■ Sleep disturbances.
■ Use of aids to sleep, such as medications or nighttime routines.

Individuals at Risk

Some individuals are at increased risk for problems in this area. Be sensitive to cues when assessing individuals with any of the following characteristics:

- Shift-work job.
- Daytime boredom and inactivity.
- Unrelieved pain.
- Restless leg syndrome.
- Nocturia.
- Anxiety.
- Depression.
- New parents.
- Teenagers.
- Cardiac or respiratory patients with dyspnea.
- Poststroke patients.
- Working parents.
- Home caregivers.

Assessment Items

History
- Generally feel rested and ready for daily activities after sleep?
- Sleep onset problems? Sleep aids used? (If you suspect a sleep problem, see Sleep Pattern Disturbance Tool below.)
- Dreams or night awakening?
- Snoring? Headache when awakening?
- Ever doze off for a second while driving? When stopped at a light or stopped in traffic? Dozing during the day? (If yes, see Epworth Daytime Sleepiness Scale at the end of this tab; if a problem, refer to physician for sleep apnea evaluation.)
- Usual bedtime? Bedtime routines?
- Rest-relaxation periods during the day or evening?

Examination
- In hospital: Observe sleep pattern and physical appearance when awake

Diagnostic Categories

The following nursing diagnoses from the NANDA International Taxonomy II (2007) describe diagnostic judgments. Blue type indicates diagnoses developed by the author, not yet reviewed by NANDA, but found useful in clinical practice (Gordon, 2006).

- **Sleep Deprivation:** Prolonged periods of time (2 to 3 days or more) without sleep (sustained natural, periodic suspension of relative unconsciousness).
- **Insomnia:** Disruption in the amount and quality of sleep that impairs functioning.

SLEEP/
REST

- **Delayed Sleep Onset:** Inability to sleep after 30 minutes when the expectation is that sleep will occur.
- **Sleep Pattern Reversal:** Change in sleep-wake cycle from nighttime sleep to predominantly daytime sleep.
- **Readiness for Enhanced Sleep:** Pattern of natural, periodic suspension of consciousness that provides adequate rest, sustains a desired lifestyle, and can be strengthened.

Family Assessment

Healthy patterns of sleep and rest are learned in the family, but not all sleep problems arise from familial factors. Environmental factors such as sleeping arrangements, sleep interruptions, and outside noises can interfere with the sleep patterns of family members. The family pattern of sleep, rest, and relaxation includes:

- Quality and quantity of members' sleep.
- Energy level.
- Use of sleep aids.
- Nighttime routines.

Families at Risk

Some families are at increased risk for problems in the sleep-rest pattern. Be sensitive to cues when assessing families with any of the following characteristics:

- Disorganized lifestyle.
- Living in overcrowded housing.
- Member who does shift work.
- Nocturnal neighborhood activity.

Assessment Items

History

- Most days, do family members seem to be well rested and ready for school and work?
- Regularity of family sleep pattern?
- Sufficient space? Quiet, dark sleeping space available?
- Young baby in family? Toddler asking to sleep in parents' bed?
- Family members find time to relax before sleep?

Examination

- If opportunity available: Observe sleeping space and arrangements.
- Family members appear alert and well rested?

No family diagnoses have been identified in this pattern.

Community Assessment

Communities have patterns of sleeping, resting, and relaxation. Some towns are said to never shut down, whereas others seem deserted in the evening. Assessment focuses on environmental factors that can interfere with sleep and rest. When assessing the community, keep these points in mind:

- Factors disturbing a community sleep-rest pattern can be obtained from residents.
- Observation of the community will reveal whether the environment is conducive to sleep and relaxation.
- Policies and regulations can be reviewed regarding noise pollution in industrial communities.

Communities at Risk

Some communities are at increased risk for problems in this area. Be sensitive to cues when assessing communities with any of the following characteristics:

- Housing built along a major highway or busy city street.
- Housing built near an airport or late-closing commercial area.

Assessment Items

History (Community Representatives)
- Generally quiet at night in most neighborhoods?
- Usual business hours? "Round-the-clock" industry?

Examination
- Activity-noise levels in business and residential districts?
- Noise regulations or laws?
- Areas where elderly people can rest when shopping, such as chairs or benches?

Diagnostic Categories

No community diagnoses have been identified in this pattern.

SLEEP/
REST

Tips for Assessing This Pattern

- When there are time pressures, screen this pattern with observation and the question: Do you generally feel rested and ready for daily activities after sleep?
- *Delayed Sleep Onset related to Anxiety* and *Sleep Deprivation related to Acute Pain* are common NANDA diagnoses. Note the problem is from the Sleep-Rest Pattern, and the reason for the problem is from another pattern.
- Pain can interfere with sleep, and sleep deprivation can increase the sensitivity to pain.
- Snoring may be a sign of sleep apnea and can produce sleep deprivation in the sleep partner. Daytime drowsiness, auto accidents due to falling asleep, and other problems can also be caused by sleep apnea.
- Listen when elderly people report insomnia. It is a myth that older people need less sleep. Lack of adequate sleep has been associated with decreased immune function, relationship disturbances, depression, hypertension, diminished alertness, and falls (Cole, 2007).
- The Environmental Protection Agency recommends hospital noise levels, on average, should not exceed 35 dB (decibels) at night.

In-Depth Assessment Tools

Sleep Pattern Disturbance Tool

Place a check in the blanks if the statement applies to you.
____Only time that I have to think is when I get into bed.
____I am quite active getting things done 2–3 hours before bed.
____I eat supper after 7:30 p.m.
____I smoke in the bedroom.
____I have an alcoholic drink before bedtime.
____My bedroom tends to be noisy.
____My bed-partner snores.
____Window shades do not darken the bedroom.
____My mattress is not really comfortable.
____Temperature in bedroom is too cold or hot.
____I have a glass of warm milk before bedtime.
____I like to watch TV in bed.
____I like to read before going to sleep.
____I get up to go to the toilet at night.
____I seem to need an hour nap in the afternoon.
____I tend to watch the clock when I cannot sleep.

____I toss and turn for over an hour or more.
____I doze a bit after meals in the daytime.
____My joints ache when I go to bed.
____My legs seem to jump when I am trying to sleep.
____I have trouble breathing in bed.
____My heart pounds sometimes, and it is scary.

From Chesson AL, Anderson WM, Littner M, et al (1999). Practice parameters for the nonpharmacologic treatment of chronic insomnia. Sleep 22(8), 1–5, with permission.

Epworth Daytime Sleepiness Scale*

This scale can be used if you suspect a sleep problem and to gauge its extent. It can either be filled out by the patient or read to him or her. The last two items, when rated as a chance, require counseling and referral.
How likely are you to doze off or fall asleep in the following situations, in contrast to feeling just tired? Use the following scale to choose the most appropriate number for each situation:

- 0: Would never doze
- 1: Slight chance of dozing
- 2: Moderate chance of dozing
- 3: High chance of dozing

Situation
____Sitting and reading
____Watching TV
____Sitting inactive in a public place (e.g., theater or a meeting)
____As a passenger in a car for an hour without a break
____Lying down to rest in the afternoon when circumstances permit
____Sitting and talking to someone
____Sitting quietly after a lunch without alcohol
____In a car while stopped for a few minutes in traffic
____Driving alone on a monotonous highway for an hour

*Scoring
- <10 points = Probably normal
- 10–12 points = Mild sleepiness
- 13–17 points = Moderate sleepiness
- 18–24 points = Severe sleepiness

Adapted from Institute for Clinical Systems Improvement, 2007 (www.icsi.org)

Cognitive-Perceptual Pattern

With the cognitive-perceptual pattern, assessment moves toward topics considered more personal. Rapport established during assessment of the previous five patterns should provide a comfortable setting for further assessment.

The cognitive-perceptual pattern describes the:

- Ability to collect and use information from the environment.
- Decision-making and other cognitive processes of individuals, families, and communities.

The neurological system is the major biological support system for this pattern and, therefore, the pattern is affected by this system's pathology.

Why This Pattern Is Important

The following are reasons that individuals, families, and communities require assessment of this pattern:

- Perception of severe discomfort, or pain, signals possible tissue damage.
- Pain interferes with life activities and results in stress and anxiety.
- Hospital and other health-care accreditation by the Joint Commission on Accreditation of Healthcare Organizations (JCAHO) includes
- Identification and treatment of pain is one important criterion of quality care delivery used in accreditation of hospitals and other health-care agencies. JCAHO reviews the documentation of pain assessment during accreditation.
- Perception is a protective mechanism and alerts the person to unsafe conditions. Cognitive-perceptual impairments interfere with this protective mechanism.
- Vision, hearing, touch, and other perceptual modalities contribute to enjoyment of people, relationships, and appreciation of the world and its beauty.
- Perception provides information used in higher cognitive processes that provide the basis for action.
- Assessment of level of consciousness, orientation, memory, reality-based thinking, and judgment guide nursing decisions about a patient's level of dependency and ability to learn. Nursing documentation about these capabilities is used when ethical dilemmas arise regarding a patient's decision-making ability.
- Data about a person's knowledge level and judgment capability are used in health teaching.

Individual Assessment

The cognitive-perceptual pattern focuses on the person's ability to collect information from the environment and use it in reasoning and other thought processes. Included are:

- Adequacy of vision, hearing, taste, touch, kinesthesia, and smell.
- Compensations or prostheses currently used, such as glasses and hearing aids.
- Pain and how it is managed.
- Cognitive functional abilities, such as orientation, memory, reasoning, judgment, and decision making.

Individuals at Risk

Some individuals are at increased risk for problems in this area. Be sensitive to cues when assessing individuals with any of the following characteristics:

- Familial history of glaucoma.
- Age:
  - Vision: ≥40 years.
  - Hearing: ≥60 years.
  - Smell, touch, kinesthesia: ≥70 years.
- African descent (vision).
- Excessive noise exposure, such as in the workplace or loud music.
- Circulatory problem.
- Trauma or surgical incisional pain.
- Cardiac or chest pain.
- Arthritis or joint pain.
- Burns.
- Cancer.
- Dementia, Alzheimer's disease, and other neurological degenerative diseases.
- Hypoxia.
- Taking medications affecting cerebral function.

Assessment Items

History
- Discomfort or pain? (If present, describe intensity using Wong-Baker Faces Pain Rating Scale, Numeric Rating Scale, or Descriptive Rating Scale below.)
- Location? Quality? When occurs? When started? What makes it worse?
- What seems to help when this occurs? Effective most of the time?

COGNITIVE PERCEPT

- Difficulty in vision or reading?
- Wear glasses? Last time vision checked? Bring glasses with you?
- Use contact lens?
- Difficulty hearing? If yes: Use hearing aid? Use frequently?
- Exposed to loud noise or music?
- Changes in taste of food?
- Changes in sense of smell?
- Changes in feeling or touch in toes, feet, hands?
- Change in memory? If yes, recent things? Things from the past? How do changes interfere with activities? If suspect memory impairment, ask today's date, day of the week, current President of the United States of America, and name of present location.
- Problems concentrating? If yes: Feel this interferes with tasks or work?
- Decisions easy or difficult to make? If difficult, ask patient to describe the difficulty. (If impaired judgment and decision making is suspected, see Judgment and Decision-Making Scale below.)
- Difficulty learning?
- Easiest way for you to learn? What helps?
- Level of school completed?

Examination

Orientation to time, including day and date; place currently in; and person, nurse or other.

Level of consciousness. (See Level of Consciousness Classification below.) If the patient is not alert, see Glasgow Coma Scale and Four Score Coma Measurement Scale below.

- Whisper test in right and left ears.
- Reads newsprint (vision).
- Can pick up a pencil (touch, kinesthesia, and fine-motor skill).
- Grasps ideas and questions during assessment; determines if abstract or concrete thinking.
- Language spoken.
- Attention span: ability to concentrate: average, short span, easily distracted.
- Understanding of verbal message: Comprehends always, sometimes, or rarely.

Diagnostic Categories

The following nursing diagnoses from the NANDA International Taxonomy II (2007) describe diagnostic judgments. Blue type indicates diagnoses developed by the author, not yet reviewed by NANDA, but found useful in clinical practice (Gordon, 2006).

- **Acute Pain (Specify Type and Location):** Verbal or coded report of the presence of indicators of severe discomfort (pain) with a duration of less than 6 months (specify type and location: joint pain, low back, cervical, knee pain).
- **Chronic Pain (Specify Type and Location):** Severe discomfort (pain) with a duration of more than 6 months (specify type and location: joint pain, low back, cervical, knee pain).
- **Pain Self-Management Deficit (Acute, Chronic):** Lack of use or insufficient use of techniques to reduce pain, such as pain medication, timing, positioning, and distraction.
- **Readiness for Enhanced Comfort:** A pattern of ease, relief, and transcendence in physical, psychospiritual, environmental, or social dimensions that can be strengthened.
- **Disturbed Sensory Perception (Specify Visual, Auditory, Kinesthetic, Gustatory, Tactile, Olfactory):** Change in the amount or patterning of incoming stimuli accompanied by a diminished, exaggerated, distorted, or impaired response to such stimuli.
- **Uncompensated Sensory Loss (Specify Type and Degree):** Uncompensated decrease in visual, hearing, touch, smell, or kinesthetic acuity.
- **Sensory Overload:** Environmental stimuli greater than habitual level of input or monotonous environmental stimuli.
- **Sensory Deprivation:** Reduced environmental and social stimuli relative to habitual (or basic orienting) level.
- **Unilateral Neglect:** Perceptually unaware of and inattentive to one side of the body and environment.
- **Deficient Knowledge (Specify Area):** Inability to state or explain information or demonstrate a required skill related to disease-management procedures, practices, or self-care health management (specify area).
- **Readiness for Enhanced Knowledge:** Presence or acquisition of cognitive information related to a specific topic is sufficient for meeting health-related goals and can be strengthened.
- **Disturbed Thought Processes (Specify):** Disruption in cognitive operations or activities, relative to chronological age expectation (specify type of alteration, as this is a broad taxonomic category).
- **Attention-Concentration Deficit:** Inability to sustain a focal awareness.
- **Acute Confusion:** Abrupt onset of global, transient changes and disturbances in attention, cognition, psychomotor activity, level of consciousness, and sleep-wake cycle.
- **Risk for Acute Confusion:** At risk for reversible disturbances of consciousness, attention, cognition, and perception that develop over a short period of time.
- **Chronic Confusion:** Irreversible long-standing or progressive deterioration of intellect and personality, characterized by decreased ability to interpret environmental stimuli and decreased capacity for intellectual thought

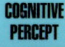

COGNITIVE PERCEPT

processes, and manifested by disturbances of memory, orientation, and behavior.

- **Impaired Environmental Interpretation Syndrome:** Consistent lack of orientation to person, place, time, or circumstances over more than 3 to 6 months that necessitates a protective environment.
- **Impaired Memory:** Inability to remember or recall bits of information or behavioral skills. Impaired memory may be attributed to pathophysiological or situational causes that are either temporary or permanent.
- **Risk for Cognitive Impairment:** Presence of risk factors for impairment in memory, reasoning, ability, judgment, and decision making.
- **Readiness for Enhanced Decision Making:** Pattern of choosing courses of action that is sufficient for meeting short- and long-term health-related goals and can be strengthened.
- **Decisional Conflict (Specify):** Uncertainty about course of action to be taken when choice among competing actions involves risk, loss, or challenge to personal life values. (Specify focus of conflict, such as surgery, therapy, abortion, divorce, or other life events.)

Family Assessment

The decisions that families make affect all functional health patterns. The same is true for communities. Decisions made by governing bodies influence the health and lives of individuals and families. Assessment of this pattern focuses on how decisions are made.

- Family patterns of problem solving and decision making.
- Information and information-gathering strategies.
- Consideration of consequences of decisions for all members.
- Future-oriented planning.

Rarely is there an opportunity at an initial home visit to talk to the whole family at once; thus, assessment data are collected from one adult family member.

This pattern describes family judgment and decision-making patterns. It includes which members participate in decisions, if consequences of decisions are considered, use of resources, and if decisions are oriented to the present or future.

Families at Risk

Some families are at increased risk for problems in this area. Be sensitive to cues when assessing families with any of the following characteristics:

- Low past opportunity to learn problem-solving skills.
- Non–English-speaking.

- Member with neurological or psychiatric disorder.
- Insufficient income for visual or hearing aids.
- Present-oriented planning.

Assessment Items

History
- Family member with visual or hearing problems? How managed?
- Important family decisions made in the last few years? How made? Members involved?

Examination
- Language spoken?
- Grasp of ideas and questions, both abstract and concrete?

Diagnostic Categories

No family diagnoses have been identified in this pattern.

Community Assessment

Public health policies reflect the important decisions a community makes in:
- Health.
- Economics.
- Education.
- Environment.
- Access to and availability of health care.
- Disaster and emergency management.

The focus of community assessment is on how decisions are made and implemented. Information is obtained through conversations with:
- Families in the community.
- Government representatives.
- Board of health.
- Representatives of industry and health-care agencies.

This is supplemented by reading government reports and community newspapers.

Communities at Risk

Some communities are at increased risk for problems in this area. Be sensitive to cues when assessing communities with any of the following characteristics:

COGNITIVE PERCEPT

- Transitioning from one ethnic or income group to another.
- Low education budget.
- Lack of facilities for psychiatric and degenerative neurological conditions, such as Alzheimer's disease, relative to community need.

Assessment Items

History (Community Representatives)

The following items are suggested for assessing the community pattern:

- Most groups speak English? Other predominant language?
- Average educational level of people in the community?
- Schools seen as good or need improving?
- Adult education desired? Available?
- Types of problems that require community decisions? Decision-making process?
- Best way to get things accomplished or changed in the community?

Examination (Community Records)

- Quality, number, and location of school facilities?
- School drop-out rate?
- Adult education programs?
- Approximate percentage of residents speaking English?
  - If high percentage: Available English as Second Language (ESL) classes?
- Government structure and decision-making lines, including organizational charts that show how decisions that affect health-care services are made?

Diagnostic Categories

No community diagnoses have been identified in this pattern.

Tips for Assessing This Pattern

- A smooth transition from the discussion about sleep to the cognitive-perceptual pattern might be: "Everyone needs a good night's sleep to feel ready for the day's activities; any pain or discomfort when you get up or at any other time?"
- Look for a pattern, not isolated behavior. Everyone at times forgets things, makes incorrect statements or poor decisions.
- Keep a piece of newsprint in your pocket to test vision.
- Look for compensations when memory or decision making starts to deteriorate. Many people try to hide early deficits so family and friends will not know.

- Self-denial occurs when changes cause anxiety. Recognize that it is very frightening to perceive mental changes in oneself or to recognize the beginning of vision or hearing loss.
- Any problem the patient describes during assessment may be used to measure reasoning, judgment, and problem-solving ability.
- Disorientation and confusion may occur in the elderly when there is some loss of vision or hearing. Watch for this change, particularly in the evening.

In-Depth Assessment Tools

Wong-Baker Faces Pain Rating Scale

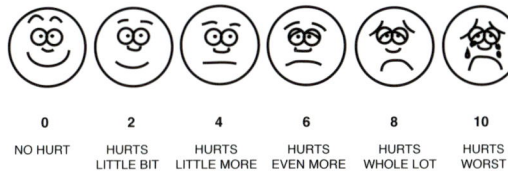

0	2	4	6	8	10
NO HURT	HURTS LITTLE BIT	HURTS LITTLE MORE	HURTS EVEN MORE	HURTS WHOLE LOT	HURTS WORST

Explain to the patient that each face is for a person who feels happy because he has no pain (hurt) or sad because he has some or a lot of pain. Face 0 is very happy because he does not hurt at all. Face 4 hurts a little more. Face 6 hurts even more. Face 8 hurts a whole lot. Face 10 hurts as much as you can imagine, although you do not have to be crying to feel this bad. Ask the person to choose the face that best describes how he or she is feeling. This rating scale is recommended for persons age 3 years and older.

Other Pain-Rating Scales

The following pain-rating scales can also be used with patients.

Numeric Rating Scale

Ask the patient to rate his or her pain on a scale from 0 (no pain) to 10 (worst pain).

0 1 2 3 4 5 6 7 8 9 10

Source: From Hockenberry MJ, Wilson D, Winkelstein ML: Wong's Essentials of Pediatric Nursing, ed. 7, St. Louis, 2005, p. 1259. Used with permission. Copyright, Mosby.

COGNITIVE PERCEPT

Descriptive Rating Scale

Ask the patient to rate pain by selecting the descriptor that he or she feels best represents the current pain level:

- No pain
- Annoying
- Uncomfortable
- Dreadful
- Horrible
- Agonizing

Identifying Areas of Referred Pain

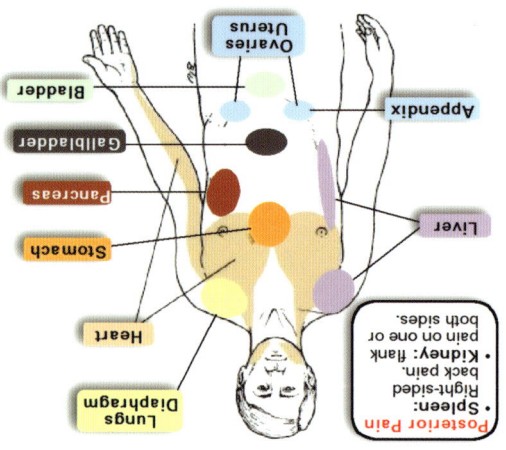

Heart · Diaphragm · Lungs · Stomach · Pancreas · Gallbladder · Bladder · Ovaries · Uterus · Appendix · Liver

Posterior Pain
- **Spleen:** Right-sided back pain.
- **Kidney:** flank pain on one or both sides.

Factors Influencing Pain

When assessing a patient with chronic pain, use the following checklist to help elicit a comprehensive description of influencing factors. This assessment can identify factors enhancing the pain and be a focus for teaching pain management.

To help you manage your pain, let us go through this list and discuss things that influence the pain and discomfort you are experiencing.

Things that start the pain:
_____

Time of day that pain is worst:
_____

Body position that makes pain worse:
_____

Activities that seem to make pain worse:
_____

Meals/foods/liquids that make pain worse:
_____

Things I do that make pain worse:
_____

Things I do that make pain less:
_____

Over-the-counter drugs/lotions that make pain less:
_____

Judgment and Decision-Making Scale

The data for assessing judgment and decision making may have to be collected over time in some cases. Family may be able to provide information.

Grade	Classification	Description
0	Independent	Decisions are consistent, reasonable, safe.
1	Modified independence	Some difficulty in new situations.
2	Minimally impaired	In specific situations, decisions become poor or unsafe and cues/supervision necessary at those times.
3	Moderately impaired	Decisions consistently poor or unsafe, cues/supervision required at all times.
4	Severely impaired	Never/rarely makes decisions.

Adapted from Center for Medicaid and Medicare Services (2003). *Minimum Data Set (MDS), Version 3.0.* April 4, 2003.

COGNITIVE PERCEPT

Level of Consciousness Classification

Determine level of consciousness on the basis of the individual's best eye, verbal, and motor response to stimuli during an interaction. The following is a method of classifying the assessment data.

Classification	Description
Alert	Awake and aware of normal external and internal stimuli. Able to interact in a meaningful way with the nurse.
Lethargy or somnolence	Not fully alert. Tends to drift to sleep when not stimulated, diminished spontaneous physical movement, loses train of thought, ideas wander.
Obtundation	Transitional stage between lethargy and stupor; difficult to arouse, meaningful testing futile, requires constant stimulation to elicit response.
Stupor or semicoma	Mumbles or groans in response to persistent and vigorous physical stimulation.
Coma	Cannot be aroused. No behavioral response to stimuli.

Assessing cognitive function. In Mezey, et al, Geriatric Nursing Protocols for Best Practice, 2nd ed. New York: Springer.

Glasgow Coma Scale

This is a widely used scoring system to quantify level of consciousness after brain injury. Document as E_V_M_; for example, E4V5M6.

Eyes open	■ Spontaneously. . . . . 4 ■ To command . . . . 3 ■ To pain. . . . . 2 **E** ■ Unresponsive. 1	Findings
Best verbal response	■ Oriented . . . . 5 ■ Confused . . . . 4 ■ Inappropriate . . . . 3 ■ Incomprehensible . . . . 2 **V** ■ Unresponsive. 1	Findings
Best motor response	■ Obeys commands . . . . 6 ■ Localizes pain. . . . . 5 ■ Withdraws from pain. . . . . 4 ■ Abnormal flexion . . . . 3 ■ Abnormal extension . . . . 2 **M** ■ Unresponsive. 1	Findings

Total_____

Four Score Coma Measurement Scale

This measure provides information on respiration not evaluated in the Glasgow scale.

Eye Response

4	Eyelids open or opened, tracking or blinking to command
3	Eyelids open but not tracking
2	Eyelids closed but open to loud voice
1	Eyelids closed but open to pain
0	Eyelids remain closed with pain

Motor Response

4	Thumbs up, fist, or peace sign to command
3	Localizing to pain
2	Flexion response to pain
1	Extensor posturing
0	No response to pain or generalized myoclonus status epilepticus

Brainstem Reflexes

4	Pupil and corneal reflexes present
3	One pupil wide and fixed
2	Pupil or corneal reflexes absent
1	Pupil and corneal reflexes absent
0	Absent pupil, corneal, and cough reflex

Respiration

4	Not intubated, regular breathing pattern
3	Not intubated, Cheyne-Stokes breathing pattern
2	Not intubated, irregular breathing pattern
1	Breathes above ventilator rate
0	Breathes at ventilator rate or apnea

From Wijdicks, et al, 2005, with permission.

COGNITIVE PERCEPT

Self-Perception–Self-Concept Pattern

The focus of assessment in the self-perception/self-concept pattern is on subjective thoughts, feelings, and attitudes about oneself. Perceptions that make up self-concept have interested philosophers and scientists for many centuries. This personal awareness has been described in its many dimensions as:

- **Self-identity:** This is the body boundary that defines the person, distinguishing the self from nonself. Name is important in identity.
- **Self-esteem or self-worth:** These are the thoughts and feelings that comprise self-evaluation, or the self-portrait of oneself.
- **Self-competency:** This is the self-evaluation of capabilities: cognitive, social, and physical.
- **Body image:** This is the mental picture of one's body related to appearance and function.
- In addition, this pattern is focused on feeling and mood states, such as:
  - Happiness
  - Anxiety
  - Hope
  - Power
  - Anger
  - Fear
  - Depression
  - Control

Each mood state is seen in health care, and each dimension of the self can be influenced by health and illness.

Why This Pattern Is Important

The following are reasons that individuals, families, and communities require assessment of this pattern:

- Severe fear or anxiety before surgery increases surgical risk.
- Leaving the protective hospital environment or facing home-care responsibilities can produce fear or anxiety at discharge if the patient is not prepared to manage his or her own care.
- Fear and anxiety are common when individuals or families are awaiting diagnosis.
- The physiological component of emotional reactions is increased heart rate and blood pressure, which is detrimental in some cardiac conditions.
- Feelings of having no control over a situation can immobilize a person and lower self-esteem.
- A family atmosphere of respect and positive regard develops and maintains members' self-esteem.

- Depression among heart attack survivors can persist for a year after leaving the hospital (Thombs, Bass, and Ford, 2006, p. 30).
- Loneliness and depression are frequently overlooked in elderly who live alone.
- Transient, reactive depression is common after a loss, disability, or onset of chronic illness.
- Families and communities can slip into feelings of hopelessness, powerlessness, and a negative vision for the future.

Individual Assessment

The self-perception–self-concept pattern describes the individual's:
- Self-identity, esteem, and image.
- Self-competency.
- Mood state.

Subjective states, such as these, require subjective assessment data for identification.

Individuals at Risk

Some individuals are at increased risk for problems in this area. Be sensitive to cues when assessing individuals with any of the the following characteristics:
- Uncertainty regarding diagnosis or surgery.
- Separation.
- Significant personal loss.
- Abandonment.
- Chronic pain.
- Forced relocation.
- History of abuse or neglect.
- Loss of body part or function.
- History of alcoholism or drug abuse.

Assessment Items

History
- We all have an idea of ourselves. How would you describe yourself?
- Most of the time feel good or not so good about yourself?
- Changes in your body or the things you can do? Are these a problem for you?
- Changes in way you feel about yourself or your body since illness started?

- Find things frequently make you angry? Annoyed? Fearful? Anxious? (If indicated, see Assessing Fears About Death below.)
- Depressed? What helps when this happens? (See manifestations of depression in the elderly at the end of this tab.)
- Ever feel you lose hope?
- Ever feel you are not able to control things in life? What helps?

Examination
- Eye contact?
- Confident manner in speech and appearance (use more than one encounter)?
- Posture?
- Dress?
- Grooming?
- Attention span? On a scale of 1 to 10, with 1 being attentive and 10 being distracted.
- Mood? On a scale of 1 to 10, with 1 being relaxed and 10 being nervous.
- Response style? On a scale of 1 to 10, with 1 being assertive and 10 being passive.
- Interaction with family members or others, if present?

Diagnostic Categories

The following nursing diagnoses from the NANDA International Taxonomy II (2007) describe diagnostic judgments. Blue type indicates diagnoses developed by the author, not yet reviewed by NANDA, but found useful in clinical practice (Gordon, 2006).

- **Fear (Specify Focus):** Feeling of dread related to an identifiable source that is perceived as a threat or danger to the self (specify focus, such as prognosis, surgical outcome, death, disability).
- **Anxiety:** Vague, uneasy feeling of discomfort or dread; the source is often nonspecific or unknown to the individual.
- **Mild Anxiety:** Increased level of arousal associated with expectation of a threat (unfocused) to the self or significant relationships.
- **Moderate Anxiety:** Increased level of arousal with selective attention and associated with expectation of a threat (unfocused) to the self or significant relationships.
- **Severe Anxiety (Panic):** Extreme arousal and scattered focus associated with expectation of a threat to the self or significant relationships.
- **Anticipatory Anxiety (Mild, Moderate, Severe):** Increased level of arousal associated with a perceived future threat (unfocused) to the self or significant relationships.
- **Death Anxiety:** Vague, uneasy feeling of discomfort or dread generated by perceptions of a real or imagined threat to one's existence.

- **Reactive Depression (Specify Situation):** Acute decrease in self-esteem, worth, or competency linked to a situational threat (specify situational threat, such as health outcome, disability, physical deterioration).
- **Risk for Loneliness:** Risk for experiencing discomfort associated with a desire or need for more contact with others.
- **Hopelessness:** Perception of limited or no alternatives or personal choices available and unable to mobilize energy on own behalf.
- **Readiness for Enhanced Hope:** A pattern of expectations and desires that is sufficient for mobilizing energy on one's own behalf and can be strengthened.
- **Powerlessness (Severe, Moderate, Low):** Perceived lack of control over a situation and perception that own actions will not significantly affect an outcome.
- **Risk for Powerlessness:** At risk for perceived lack of control over a situation or ability to significantly affect an outcome.
- **Readiness for Enhanced Power:** A pattern of participating knowingly in change that is sufficient for well-being and can be strengthened.
- **Risk for Compromised Human Dignity:** At risk for perceived loss of respect and honor.
- **Chronic Low Self-Esteem:** Long-standing negative self-evaluation or feelings about self or self-capabilities, which may be directly or indirectly expressed.
- **Situational Low Self-Esteem:** Development of a negative perception of self-worth in response to a situation.
- **Risk for Situational Low Self-Esteem:** Presence of risk factors for developing a negative perception of self-worth in response to a current situation (specify).
- **Readiness for Enhanced Self-Concept:** Pattern of perception or ideas about the self that is sufficient for well-being and can be strengthened.
- **Disturbed Body Image:** Negative feelings or perceptions about characteristics, function, or limits of body or body part.
- **Disturbed Personal Identity:** Inability to distinguish between self and nonself.
- **Risk for Self-Directed Violence:** Presence of risk factors for behavior that can be physically, emotionally, or sexually harmful to the self.

Family Assessment

The family self-perception–self-concept pattern focuses on family identity, self-esteem, self-confidence, image, and mood state. Family identity includes the following forms:

- **Nuclear family:** Parents and children.

- **Extended family:** Relatives in distant geographic areas.
- **Blended family:** Second marriage, in which the husband and wife have children from previous marriages that blend with children from the current marriage.

A household of nonrelated persons living together may also refer to each other as family because of the supportive network provided. Family self-esteem is based on the:

- Quality of relationships.
- Cohesion of members.
- Concern for each other.

Family self-competency is the capability to handle:

- Daily activities.
- Financial matters.
- Plans for the future.
- Family stress.

Families at Risk

Some families are at increased risk for problems in this area. Be sensitive to cues when assessing the self-perception–self-concept pattern of families or groups with any of the following characteristics:

- Financial difficulties.
- Drug abuse.
- Alcohol abuse.
- Homelessness.
- Member of a minority cultural group in the community.

Assessment Items

History

- Family members living at home?
- Extended family in close touch? (Diagram relationships if relevant; see genogram below.)
- Most of time family members feel good or not so good about themselves as a family?

Examination

- General mood of family? Happy? Anxious? Depressed?
- What helps improve family mood?
- General mood state? On a scale of 1 to 10, with 1 being relaxed and 10 being nervous.
- Members' response style? On a scale of 1 to 10, with 1 being passive and 10 being assertive.

Constructing a Family Genogram

A genogram allows you to identify familial risk factors at a glance. When developing a genogram, use symbols to represent family members, and include a key to explain the symbols.

Circle if in the household:

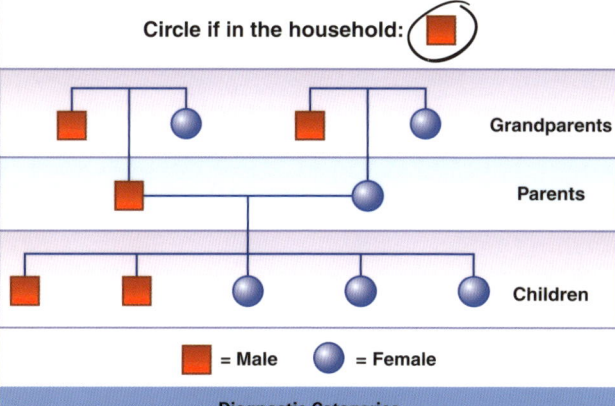

		Grandparents
		Parents
		Children

■ = Male ● = Female

Diagnostic Categories

No family diagnoses have been identified in this pattern.

Community Assessment

The self-perception–self-concept pattern describes community members' perceptions of the community self-image, identity, and stability. It includes the amount of cultural, age, racial, and socioeconomic diversity of the community and the general attitude toward minority groups within the community.

Communities at Risk

Some communities are at increased risk for problems in this area. Be sensitive to cues when assessing communities with any of the following characteristics:

- High crime rates, including against property.
- Littering of streets.
- Nonmaintained property.
- Changing demographics.
- Racial or ethnic tension.
- Unemployment.
- Teen suicide.
- School bullying.

Assessment Items

History (Community Representatives)

- Good community to live in? Why?
- Status going up, down, or staying about the same?
- Old community? Fairly new?
- Does any age group predominate?
- People's mood in general: Enjoying life? Stressed? Feeling down?
- People generally have the kinds of abilities needed in this community?
- Community or neighborhood functions? Parades? Picnics?

Examination

- Racial, ethnic mix, if appropriate.
- Socioeconomic levels.
- General observations of mood: people in the community and at meetings.
- Suicide rate by age groups.
- Available mental health services relative to need.

Diagnostic Categories

No community diagnoses have been identified in this pattern.

Tips for Assessing This Pattern

- Keep in mind that mood states, such as anxiety and anger, can be conta-gious in a family or in a community. Feelings and attitudes, such as hopelessness and powerlessness, are also communicated indirectly.
- Subgroups within the community can also feel powerless and feel they lack control over issues they believe influence their lives, such as a group of immigrants wanting a translator available 24 hours per day in the local emergency room.

- An individual may be experiencing fear over an impending surgery. Further assessment can elicit the meaning of the experience, such as:
  - Pain or mutilation.
  - Risk of dying.
  - Loss of control, as from anesthesia.
  - Prognosis and its effect on role and responsibilities.
- Basing judgments on assumptions versus assessment can lead to errors.
- Early assessment and intervention can prevent the development of *Chronic Low Self-Esteem,* which is a risk with:
  - Negative childhood experiences within the family or peer group.
  - Disfigurement from birth.
  - Chronic medical problem.
- The following self-negating expressions of *Disturbed Body Image* after a loss of body part or body function should not be missed:
  - Worthlessness.
  - Gender identity questions.
  - Inadequacy, shame, or guilt.
  - Hopelessness.
- Distinguish between fear and anxiety. Interventions are different. Fear is focused; anxiety is diffuse.

In-Depth Assessment Tools

Assessing Fears About Death

The following is a list of fears and concerns people have when they are terminally ill. Before assessing a patient who is dying, it may be useful for the nurse to review the list in order to help the patient to focus. Interventions are different for each of the items below.

Concern About Others*
- Worrying about being the cause of others' grief and suffering.
- Fear of leaving family to manage alone after death.
- Worrying about the effect of own death on significant others, including financial burden.

Concern About Self
- Fear of the process of dying.
- Powerlessness, including issues related to dying.
- Fear of loss of physical and mental abilities when dying.
- Pain related to dying.

*From NANDA International (2007), pp. 11–12.

- Concern about total loss of control over any aspect of own death.
- Fear of delayed demise.
- Fear of premature death because it prevents the accomplishment of important life goals.

After-Death Concerns
- Concern about meeting one's creator.
- Feeling doubtful about the existence of God or a higher being.
- Concern about what happens to "me" after death.

Detection of Depression in the Elderly

Risk Factors for Depression in Elderly

- Lack of social supports.
- Physically ill.
- Stressful life events, such as death of a loved one or divorce.
- Recent loss of a spouse.
- Caregiver for spouse or other family member.
- Caregiver for grandchildren.
- Being female.
- Prior episode of major depression.
- Family history of depressive disorders.
- History of prior suicide attempts.
- History of alcohol or substance abuse.

The manifestations of depression in the elderly are:

- Complaints of somatic (physical) rather than psychological symptoms.
- Denial of feeling sad.
- Apathy and withdrawal.
- Feelings of guilt.
- Reduced self-esteem.
- Inability to concentrate.
- Insomnia
- Memory impairment.

Adapted from National Guidelines, National Guideline Center. Used with permission from developer: University of Iowa Gerontological Nursing Intervention Research Core. School of Nursing, University of Iowa, Iowa City.

Role-Relationship Pattern

Quality of life is greatly influenced by the roles and relationships established with family, friends, or the broader community. In many cases, roles define our identity and, within each role, relationships are established. Friendships among individuals, working relationships, and family and neighborhood relationships are part of most people's lives.

This pattern focuses on roles and relationships of individuals, families, and communities that may be influenced by health-related factors or may offer support during illness.

Why This Pattern Is Important

The following are reasons that individuals, families, and communities require assessment of this pattern:

- Role functions can be a source of stress, particularly job stress.
- Work roles can be affected by chronic illness and impact income and self-image.
- The parenting role can require adjustments in other pattern areas, particularly with a first birth, premature birth, or a child with congenital problems.
- Dysfunctions in other health patterns can interfere with roles and relationships. For example:
  - Loss of a significant person (or even a pet or possession) can lead to dysfunctional grieving.
  - Activity intolerance or impaired mobility may interfere with work roles and affect family income.
  - Fatigue and activity intolerance can lead to social isolation when elderly are living alone.
  - Physical or mental illness can disrupt family roles and relationships.
  - Depression or anxiety can interfere with role functions and relationships.
- Role relationships are a source of social support that can be called upon for:
  - Instrumental support (helping by doing things).
  - Affective support (caring).
- Social support from family and friends is always important, but it is particularly needed during illness or a life crisis. It offers:
  - Acceptance and understanding.
  - Caring and sharing.
  - Validation of self-worth.
  - Companionship.

ROLE/
RELATION

- Communities make educational programs and services available to prevent:
  - Interpersonal violence.
  - Impaired parenting, including child abuse.
  - Domestic violence.
  - Unemployment.

Individual Assessment

The role-relationship pattern describes the individual's work, family, and social roles that might be affected by events or illness. Within these roles, relationships range from intimate to remote. Roles can have the following characteristics:

- Role satisfaction or dissatisfaction.
- Role performance.
- Role conflict, strain, or loss.

Also, the following factors that can place a strain on relationships are included in assessment:

- Impaired communication, such as through aphasia.
- Not speaking dominant language.
- Translocation, including immigration, moving from home to nursing home, and moving from intensive to standard care.
- Caregiving burden.
- Alcoholism or use of drugs.

Individuals at Risk

Some individuals are at increased risk for problems in their role-relationship pattern. Be sensitive to cues when assessing individuals with any of the following characteristics:

- Nonelective hospitalization.
- Isolation from family and friends during crisis.
- Language barrier.
- Loss of:
  - Significant person or pet.
  - Possession.
  - Job or status.
- Significant home care or dependent needs.
- Prolonged caregiving.
- History of antisocial violence or abuse.
- History of drug or alcohol abuse.

- Teenage or single parent.
- Homeless.

Assessment Items

History

- Live alone? Family structure?
- Problems in either the nuclear or extended family you have difficulty handling?
- How are problems usually handled?
- Family or others dependent on you? How are they managing while you are here?
  If a long-term care provider: Ever get very angry and stressed with the person you are caring for? (If suspect caregiver role strain, see the Caregiving Needs Checklist below to evaluate caregiving burden.)
- Recent losses?
- If appropriate: How are family and friends responding to your illness?
- If patient has children: Problems with children? Difficulty handling problems?
- If appropriate and if married or living with partner: How do you and your partner settle arguments?
- Do you feel safe in your current relationship? This item is designed to screen for domestic violence. Some health-care facilities require this screening. It is important that this question be asked when the partner is not present. (See Screening for Domestic Violence below for in-depth assessment.)
- Belong to social groups, such as religious groups, or clubs?
- Close friend you can confide in?
- Ever feel lonely? If yes, how often do those feelings occur?
- Things generally go well at work? School?
- Income sufficient for needs?
- Feel part of (or isolated from) the neighborhood?

Examination

- Interaction among family members or others if present.

Diagnostic Categories

The following nursing diagnoses from the NANDA International Taxonomy II (2007) describe diagnostic judgments about the individual. Blue type indicates diagnoses developed by the author, not yet reviewed by NANDA, but found useful in clinical practice (Gordon, 2006).

- **Grieving:** Normal, complex process that includes emotional, physical, spiritual, social, and intellectual responses and behaviors by which individuals, families, and communities incorporate an actual, anticipated, or perceived loss into daily life.
- **Complicated Grieving:** A disorder that occurs after the death of a significant other, in which the experience of distress accompanying bereavement fails to follow normative expectations and manifests in functional impairment.
- **Risk for Complicated Grieving:** Presence of risk factors that occur after the death of a significant other, in which the distress accompanying bereavement fails to follow normative expectations and manifests in functional impairment.
- **Anticipatory Grieving:** Expectation of loss of significant relationship; includes people, possessions, job, status, home, ideals, and parts or processes of the body.
- **Chronic Sorrow:** Cyclical, recurring, and potentially progressive pattern of pervasive sadness, experienced in response to continual loss, throughout the trajectory of a chronic illness or disability.
- **Ineffective Role Performance (Specify):** Change, conflict, denial of role responsibilities, or inability to perform role responsibilities (specify type; this is a broad taxonomic category).
- **Unresolved Independence-Dependence Conflict:** Need and desire to be dependent (or independent) with a therapeutic, maturational, or social expectation to be independent (or dependent).
- **Social Isolation or Social Rejection:** Condition of aloneness experienced by the individual and perceived as imposed by others and as a negative or threatening state.
- **Social Isolation:** Feelings of aloneness attributed to interpersonal interaction below level desired or required for personal integrity.
- **Impaired Social Interaction:** Insufficient or excessive quantity or ineffective quality of social exchange.
- **Developmental Delay: Social Skills (Specify):** Demonstrates deviation from age-group norms in acquisition of social skills.
- **Relocation Stress Syndrome:** Physiological or psychosocial disturbance following transfer from one environment to another.
- **Risk for Relocation Stress Syndrome:** Risk for physiological or psychosocial disturbance following transfer from one environment to another.
- **Impaired Parenting (Specify Impairment):** Inability of the primary caretaker to create, maintain, or regain an environment that promotes the optimal growth and development of the child.
- **Risk for Impaired Parenting (Specify):** Risk for inability of primary caretaker to create, maintain, or regain an environment that promotes the optimal growth and development of the child.

- **Parental Role Conflict.** Role confusion and conflict experienced by parents in response to crisis.
- **Weak Parent-Infant Attachment:** Pattern of nonreciprocal bonding relationship between parent and infant or primary caretaker and infant.
- **Risk for Impaired Parent-Infant/Child Attachment:** Disruption of the interactive process between parent or significant other and infant that fosters the development of a protective and nurturing reciprocal relationship.
- **Parent-Infant Separation:** Presence of factors that prohibit interaction between infant and parents.
- **Readiness for Enhanced Parenting:** Pattern of providing an environment for children or other dependent persons that is sufficient to nurture growth and development and can be strengthened.
- **Caregiver Role Strain:** Caregiver perceives difficulty in performing family caregiver role.
- **Risk for Caregiver Role Strain:** Caregiver is vulnerable for perceived difficulty in performing the family caregiver role.
- **Impaired Verbal Communication:** Reduced or absent ability to use language in human interaction.
- **Readiness for Enhanced Communication:** Pattern of exchanging information and ideas with others is sufficient for meeting needs and life goals and can be strengthened.
- **Developmental Delay: Communication Skills (Specify Type):** Demonstrates deviations from age-group norms in development of communications skills (specify type of skill).
- **Risk for Other-Directed Violence:** Behaviors in which an individual demonstrates that he or she can be physically, emotionally, or sexually harmful to others.

Family Assessment

The idea of family is defined in many ways. In some instances, friends fulfill traditional functions of family. In the traditional family, relationships vary from intimate to instrumental in the following roles:

- Parenting.
- Marital.
- Sociopolitical community.

The family role-relationship pattern focuses on family structure and processes. Ideally, a family provides an environment for individual growth and development, with attention to the following areas:

- Physical.
- Psychosocial.

Assessment of a family frequently requires:

- Moral.
- Spiritual.
- Individual assessment, if one or more members have a health problem.
- Community assessment, if a particular health or social problem is affected by the environment.

Families at Risk

Some families are at increased risk for problems in this area. Be sensitive to cues when assessing families or groups with any of the following characteristics:

- Family member with a diagnosis of degenerative, chronic disease.
- Perinatal loss.
- Death of family member.
- Immigrant family with lack of predeparture counseling or support.
- Language barrier.
- Recent retirement.
- Divorce or separation.
- History of domestic violence or abuse.
- Prolonged caregiving.

Assessment Items

The following are suggested items for assessing this pattern. If data suggest problems, further in-depth assessment will be needed. This may require a home visit.

History

- Family or household members: List ages of members and family structure (see Constructing a Family Genogram, Tab 9.)
- Current problem in either the nuclear or extended family that is difficult to handle?
- If children: Child-rearing problems? Problems guiding teenagers?
- Members respect the privacy of other family members?
- Number of meals family can eat together per day?
- Family has joint recreational activities?
- Relationships among family members? Among siblings? Between parents? Extended family?
- Members support each other?
- Income sufficient for family needs?
- Feel part of (or isolated from) community? From neighbors?
- Any adult-dependent members requiring care? Who is the caregiver? Any problems? (See Caregiving Needs Assessment below.)

Examination
- Interaction among family members, if present?
- Family leadership roles observed?

Diagnostic Categories

The following nursing diagnoses from the NANDA International Taxonomy II (2007) are used to describe diagnostic judgments.

- **Interrupted Family Processes (Specify):** Change in family relationships or functioning that is not supporting well-being of members.
- **Dysfunctional Family Process: Alcoholism:** Psychosocial, spiritual, and physiological functions of family unit are chronically disorganized, leading to conflict, denial of problems, resistance to change, ineffective problem solving, and a series of self-perpetuating crises.
- **Readiness for Enhanced Family Processes:** Pattern of family functioning that is sufficient to support the well-being of family members and can be strengthened.

Community Assessment

The role-relationship pattern focuses on roles within the community and relationships that affect health. Included are:

- Opportunities for community involvement and social activities.
- Composition of community, including ethnic, racial, and age groups.
- Relationships among ethnic, racial, and age groups.
- Resources, including natural resources, industry, and health care.
- Laws, regulations, and procedures that govern roles and relationships and give structure to society.

Communities at Risk

Some communities are at increased risk for problems in relationships. Be sensitive to cues when assessing communities with any of the following characteristics:

- History of ethnic or racial problems or violence.
- Isolation of ethnic or racial groups.
- Tense relationships among groups.
- People feeling powerless over a political issue affecting their lives.
- Lack of community or senior center.
- Lack of church or community caregiver respite programs.
- Lack of church or community bereavement programs.

- Inadequate mental health services.
- High unemployment.
- High rate of school dropout.

Assessment Items

History (Community Representatives)
- People seem to get along well together here?
- Places where people tend to go to socialize?
- People feel government hears them?
- High or low participation at community meetings?
- Enough work for everybody?
- Wages fair?
- People seem to like the kind of work available? Are they happy in their jobs?
- Problems with violence in the neighborhoods?
- Family violence? Child, spouse, or elder abuse?
- Get along with adjacent communities? Collaborate on any community projects?
- Do neighbors seem to support each other?
- Community get-togethers?

Examination
- Interactions among people, including health-related meetings?
- Statistics on personal or interpersonal violence?
- Suicide statistics by age group?
- Statistics on employment?
- Statistics on income and poverty?
- Divorce rate?

Diagnostic Categories

No community diagnoses have been identified in this pattern.

Tips for Assessing This Pattern

- Roles and relationships within community groups can be assessed by:
    - Attendance at health-related, government meetings.
    - Talking to people.
    - Looking at documents, including health regulations and reports.
    - Reading local newspapers and police reports.
    - Conducting interviews.

- An occupational history can reveal exposure to stress, accidents, or environmental contaminants.
- When assessing work stress, use open-ended questions. If warranted, follow with focused questions to obtain specific details.
- If a family has recently moved from another country, moved within a country, or left a familiar lifestyle, this may cause feelings of loss and isolation. Assess family members for the following symptoms of relocation syndrome:
  - Concerned or upset over transfer, relocation.
  - Feeling of powerlessness or anger regarding the move, if did not choose to move.
  - Sleep or eating disturbances.
  - Anxiety, apprehension.

Confusion or increased mortality is a risk if elderly moved within and between nursing homes against wishes.

- Nonverbal messages are an important aspect of communication. Give attention to the person's body language and speech characteristics as well as to the words.
- A genogram is useful when encountering:
  - Complex family structure.
  - Support system deficit.
  - Family problems.
- When assessing marital, sibling, parent-child, patient–care provider relationships, observe a few interactions over time before making an inference. This avoids errors. An exception to this rule is when you assess threats of violence or abuse.

In-Depth Assessment Tools

Caregiving Needs Checklist

The following is a listing of possible caregiving needs in the home. Assess pre-discharge or at a home visit or a nursing home. Check items requiring either assistance from another person (A) or supervision (S).

Eating

____Food shopping: Transportation, selecting, and carrying
____Preparing and cooking food; use of stove
____Eating: Bringing food from receptacle to mouth
____Opening containers, picking up utensils or cup

Dressing and Grooming

___ Shopping: Clothes
___ Choosing clothing (decision making)
___ Putting on/taking off clothing; upper and lower body
___ Shaving or applying makeup

Bathing—Hygiene

___ Getting to water source, such as shower or tub
___ Washing body using bath supplies
___ Regulating bath water and temperature
___ Drying body

Toileting

___ Getting to toilet or commode; sitting or rising
___ Flushing toilet; emptying commode
___ Manipulating clothing
___ Performing proper toilet hygiene

Home Management

___ Cleaning: Light
___ Cleaning: Heavy
___ Laundry
___ Repairs and maintenance
___ Shopping: Supplies, replacement of household goods

Personal Finances

___ Paying bills and taxes
___ Monitoring checking account; writing checks
___ Overseeing investments
___ Paying helpers

Organization and Communication

___ Accessing resources
___ Communicating with care providers and insurers
___ Accessing community resources, such as American Cancer Society and American Lung Association
___ Handling personal mail

Health-Related Activities

___ Taking medications as prescribed
___ Obtaining medications
___ Recognizing symptoms and complications that need medical or nursing attention
___ Seeking medical or nursing consultation when needed
___ Carrying out treatments as prescribed
___ Carrying out dressing changes

____Managing intravenous, oxygen, dialysis, and other treatments
____Making appointments for follow-up care
____Obtaining transportation to health services
____Carrying out health promotion/preventive actions related to disease; immunizations
____Organizing daily exercise program
____Managing incontinence (bowel/bladder)

Pet Care
____Feeding
____Walking
____Cleaning boxes, cages
____Grooming

Diversional Activities
____Organizing materials for hobby or diversional activity
____Going to a social event
____Ordering and reading newspaper, magazines, books

Spiritual Activities
____Attending religious services
____Obtaining transportation to services
____Arranging home religious practices
____Arranging home visit by religious representatives

Screening for Domestic Violence

Men and women may be victims or perpetrators of domestic violence in either heterosexual or same-sex relationships. Only the care provider and patient should be present during assessment, including when screening teens about their dating relationships. In a nonjudgmental manner, start with one or more of the following questions:

■ In general, how would you describe your relationship?
_____
_____

■ How do you and your partner settle arguments?
_____
_____

■ Do you feel safe in your current relationship?
_____
_____

■ Use the following listing as a way of reviewing present information about the situation and for further assessment.

ROLE/
RELATION

Injury: Examples include burns, bruises in unusual locations, facial injuries, repeated visits for minor trauma, delay in seeking treatment, injury not consistent with history.

Somatic Complaints Not Attributable to a Medical Diagnosis: Examples include insomnia, nightmares, and abdominal, pelvic, or neck pain.

Sexual Problems: Examples include pelvic inflammatory disease, sexually transmitted diseases, vaginitis, pelvic pain, and teen pregnancy.

Psychological Problems: Examples include alcohol and drug use, anxiety and panic attacks, depression, eating disorders, post-traumatic stress signs, and suicidal ideation or attempt.

Presentation: Examples include angry or anxious body language, comments about emotional abuse or a friend who is abused, flat affect, and minimizing statements.

Isolating Self From Family and Friends: Examples include not wanting to notify family about hospitalization and withdrawing from friends.

Observations: Examples include fear of partner; defers to partner to answer questions; partner hovers, appears overly concerned, will not leave patient unattended; and patient reluctant to speak in front of or to disagree with partner.

Adapted from Agency for Health Research and Quality.
Nationalguidelineclearinghouse.com.*Domestic violence Guideline,* 2006

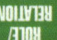

Sexuality-Reproductive Pattern

Sexuality is the behavioral expression of sexual identity. It is the:

- Perception and feeling of being male or female that develops from bio-psycho-cultural influences starting in early childhood. It is influenced by nature (genetics) and nurture (environment).
- Attraction and feelings toward members of the opposite, same, or both genders, also known as sexual orientation.

Although sexuality and sexual relationships are frequently portrayed in films, television, and advertising, individuals and families consider these topics private subjects. The importance of discussing this topic with patients needs to be clear, and judgment has to be used in determining an approach that is comfortable for the nurse and the patient. This approach includes:

- Realizing that sexuality and sexual relations are an aspect of health.
- Knowing that assessment is important because this pattern can be affected by:
  - Illness or disability.
  - Medication, such as frequently prescribed antihypertensive and antidepressant drugs.
  - Aging.
  - Recreational drugs.
- Appreciating that the approach to the subject needs to be altered for different age groups and different cultures.

Assessment of individual, family, and community sexuality-reproductive patterns *focuses on:*

- Reproductive issues and satisfaction with sexual identity and sexual relations.
- Family attitudes toward sexuality and reproduction that are communicated and become the pattern for the next generation.
- Community educational programs and standards of behavior set through political, legislative, and social action.

Why This Pattern Is Important

The following are reasons that individuals, families, and communities require assessment of this pattern:

- The incidence of AIDS in the United States is decreasing in the male homosexual population but increasing in women and heterosexual couples.
- The incidence of sexually transmitted disease (STD) is a major health problem. For example, one in four women and one in five men have

genital herpes, which is recurrent, contagious, and incurable (Gardner, 2006; Beauman, 2005). Many of these diseases have a latent phase, are asymptomatic for a time after infection, and can be transmitted even with safe sex practice.

- Infection with the human papillomavirus is difficult to cure and is implicated in cervical cancer. A vaccine is available and recommended for sexually active females, beginning at the sixth-grade level.
- Many parents need information and assistance in providing sex education to their children.
- Parents and the community need to take measures to protect children from abuse, sexual violence, and teenage pregnancy.
- Community health education programs and safety measures, such as lighting, police protection, and vigilance, are necessary to prevent rape in high-risk areas.
- Menstruation and menopause are difficult for some women. Individual responses can be influenced by biological, psychosocial, and cultural factors.
- Effects of hormonal changes in menopause need to be monitored.
- Families may need or desire health education and counseling regarding reproduction.

Individual Assessment

The expression of love and caring in a sexual relationship and creation of a family are important aspects of the sexuality-reproductive pattern. This can be interrupted by loss of a partner through death or divorce, infertility, illness, and disability. In addition, STDs, abuse, and changes due to aging affect sexual relationships. Adjustments in sexual practices are usually required with the following:

- Spinal cord injury and stroke.
- Renal disease and dialysis.
- Colostomy and other ostomies.
- Cardiopulmonary condition.
- Neurovascular (male) and hormonal (female) changes with aging.

Adjustments, such as abstinence or learning safe sex practices, are also required because of the incidence of STDs. The assessment of the individual's sexuality-reproductive pattern focuses on:

- Sexuality.
- Sexual relations.
- Reproduction.
- Family planning.
- Menstruation and menopause.

When assessing this pattern, expect to find differences in attitudes toward sexuality and sexual relationships among and within cultures and age groups. For example, you would use a different approach for a widowed, frail, 85-year-old white female than you would for an unmarried, 25-year-old, sexually active male.

Individuals at Risk

Some individuals are at increased risk for problems in this area. Be sensitive to cues when assessing individuals with any of the following characteristics:

- History of sexual abuse.
- Multiple sex partners.
- Unprotected sex.
- Marital conflict.
- Domestic violence.
- Alcohol abuse (episodic or chronic).
- Illness, such as diabetes.
- Medications, such as hypertensive medications.
- Neurovascular (male) and hormonal (female) changes of aging.
- Conflicts (social and peer pressures versus prohibitions and values).
- Body or self-image disturbance.

Assessment Items

History
- Is your sexual relationship satisfying? Problems?
- Use of medications to influence sexual performance?
- Use of safe sex practices? Always? Sometimes? Never?
- If appropriate to age: Use family planning methods? How long? Problems?
- Female: At what age did menstruation start? Last menstrual period? Problems?
- Female: Para? Gravida?

Examination
None, unless a full physical examination is indicated, in which case include pelvic examination.

Diagnostic Categories

The following nursing diagnoses from the NANDA International Taxonomy II (2007) describe judgments about the individual:

- **Ineffective Sexuality Pattern:** Expression of concern regarding own sexuality.
- **Sexual Dysfunction:** Change in sexual function, which is viewed as unsatisfying, unrewarding, or inadequate.
- **Rape Trauma Syndrome:** Sustained maladaptive response to a forced, violent sexual penetration against the victim's will and consent.
- **Rape Trauma Syndrome: Compound Reaction:** Forced, violent sexual penetration against the victim's will and consent. The trauma syndrome that develops from this attack or attempted attack includes an acute phase of disorganization of the victim's lifestyle and a long-term process of reorganization of lifestyle.
- **Rape Trauma Syndrome: Silent Reaction:** Presence of signs and symptoms but without victim's mentioning to anyone that rape has occurred.

Family Assessment

The family provides an environment for the development of healthy patterns of interaction related to sexuality and caring relationships. The family sexuality-reproductive pattern focuses on the satisfaction or dissatisfaction with:

- Marital relationship.
- Sexual relationship.
- Family planning.
- Ability to educate and counsel children in sexual matters.

As stated in Tab 10, Role-Relationship Pattern, the idea of family is defined in many ways, and many types of relationships have family characteristics. Assessment has to be tailored to the situation.

Families at Risk

Some families are at increased risk for problems in this area. Be sensitive to cues when assessing families with any of the following characteristics:

- History of domestic violence.
- Verbal abuse or humiliation (current or historical).
- Recent loss of significant other.
- Death of a child.
- Knowledge deficit regarding sex education.
- Lack of privacy.
- Stress, such as from job, family, finances, or other responsibilities.
- Chronic disease.

Assesment Items

History
- If sexual partner within household or situation: Are sexual relations satisfying? Problems?
- Elderly married: Changes in your and your partner's interest in sex?
- Unmarried: Problems regarding sex?
- Introductory question: Use of family planning?
- Using contraceptives? How long? Problems in use?
- If appropriate: Is it easy to find time and privacy for intimacy?
- If children of appropriate age: Feel comfortable in explaining or discussing sexual subjects with your children?
- If children of appropriate age: Children sexually active? Know about safe sex?

Diagnostic Categories

No family diagnoses have been identified in this pattern.

Community Assessment

Although in flux, communities have standards, both written and unwritten, for socially acceptable behavior. Social, cultural, and religious directives influence these standards. Community standards are one basis for national, state, or local laws or regulations for the following:

- Ratings for movie films.
- Selling printed or video adult material.
- Acceptability of radio and television content.
- Time when abortion permitted.
- Marriage licensing, including age allowed.
- Adult intercourse with minors or against wishes.

Assessment of the community's sexuality-reproductive pattern focuses on:

- Sex education, including education provided at schools and community programs.
- Programs to prevent sexual violence.
- Controls on adult entertainment.
- Reproductive issues (more general than local).

Communities at Risk

Some communities are at increased risk for problems in this area. Be sensitive to cues when assessing communities with any of the following characteristics:

- Increasing number of teen pregnancies.
- Few community controls on adult entertainment, including movies, bars, and bookstores.
- Insufficient crime prevention.
- Lack of rape crisis centers.
- Insufficient prevention and treatment clinics for STDs.
- High rates of divorce and single-parent households.

Assessment Items

History (Community Representatives)

- Do people feel there are problems with pornography, prostitution, or child safety, including child predators?
- Sufficient police protection to prevent sexual violence?
- In residential areas, neighborhood watch groups?
- Do people want and support sex education in schools?
- Sufficient prenatal clinic facilities?

Examination

- Average family size and number of children.
- Male-to-female ratio.
- Average maternal age.
- Maternal mortality rate.
- Infant mortality rate.
- Teen pregnancy rate.
- Divorce rate.
- Abortion rate
- Sexual violence statistics.
- Laws and regulations regarding birth control information.

Diagnostic Categories

No community diagnoses have been identified in this pattern.

Tips for Assessing This Pattern

- For a smooth transition, move from marital status in the role-relationship pattern to one of the following questions:
  - Married: Is the sexual relationship in your marriage satisfying? Problems?
  - Unmarried: Are you sexually active in any way? If yes: Problems in your sexual relations?
  - Elderly married: Changes in your and your wife or husband's interest in sex?
  - Elderly unmarried: Problems regarding sex?
- Ask screening questions in a voice and manner similar to the way other patterns are assessed to let the person know it is all right to discuss sexual concerns.
- The sexuality-reproductive pattern could be integrated into the role-relationship pattern. However, keeping it separate increases visibility and may prevent this area of health from being neglected. Reasons from around the world why this pattern is neglected by nurses include:
  - Not knowing how to ask the questions or what words to use.
  - Gender difference between nurse and patient, such as a female nurse with male patient and male nurse with female patient.
  - Fear of embarrassment if the patient asks a difficult question (possible double embarrassment from the content and not having an answer).
  - Questions are not relevant to the patient's disease (although other things not relevant are assessed).
  - Lack of time (worldwide reason).
- Recognizing the hesitancy to assess this pattern among nurses and physicians, some institutions suggest the PLISSIT Model, which specifies four levels of communication. (Katz, 2006; Annon, 1974.) The nurse chooses the most comfortable one for her or his level of expertise:
  - **P**ermission: both verbal and nonverbal message that it is acceptable to ask questions
  - **L**imited **I**nformation: Information is provided.
  - **S**pecific **S**uggestions: For the problem.
  - **I**ntensive **T**herapy: Consult sexuality specialist.
- If encountering a high rate of abortion, sexual assault, or abuse in a community, assess sexual and reproductive health education programs in schools, and obtain information from school nurses, parent-teacher associations, and police.
- Information about sexuality that patients share should not be discussed among staff or with others. Sexual orientation is usually not documented on patient record.

- When using the diagnosis *Ineffective Sexuality Pattern*, avoid superficial assessment. Assess further to identify difficulties, changes, limitations, or conflicts that may be due to any of the following:
    - Fear of acquiring an STD.
    - Fear of pregnancy.
    - Knowledge deficit about alternative responses to illness, aging, or a change in body function or structure.
    - Lack of privacy.
    - Conflict with sexual orientation or variant preferences.
    - Altered relationships with significant other (NANDA, 2007, p. 198).
- Recognize that changes in body function or structure can cause disturbances in body image that may affect sexual relationships. Examples include:
    - Obesity.
    - Mastectomy or hysterectomy.
    - Prostatectomy.
    - Myocardial infarction.
    - Changes of aging.
- Judgment has to be exercised in assessing sexual orientation. Usually, if an accepting manner has been communicated, the patient may state his or her orientation when questions around marital status or family life are asked. If not asked at this time, the decision to directly ask sexual orientation is a choice between invasion of privacy versus the effect sexual orientation can have on health risk factors, information rights, and legal issues and the resulting need for different types of health education.
- When elderly persons, cognitively impaired or not, report or manifest signs of sexual assault, assessment must follow forensic protocols and reporting laws (National Center for Elder Abuse, 2004; Burgess et al, 2005).

Coping–Stress Tolerance Pattern

Individuals, families, and communities experience stress that can lead to higher levels of function or to disorganization. Factors influencing the direction include:

- Severity of the stress.
- Type of coping responses.
- Available support systems.

Throughout life, socially acceptable, healthy coping strategies are learned. These include problem solving, relaxation, and interpersonal communication. Terms specific to stress are:

- **Stressor:** A process, event, person, or situation that produces a fight-or-flight, psycho-physiological response when a threat to self-integrity is perceived. A stressor can be acute, such as an unplanned relocation, or chronic, such as poor relationships with in-laws. There are different types of stress:
    - **Psychological stress:** Manifested as fear or anxiety, it is an autonomic response to a threatening event.
    - **Physiological stress:** A response of body systems to internal or external demands, such as what the heart and circulatory system experience during exercise.
- **Coping strategies:** Behaviors used to manage anxiety or fear related to a threatening event. Strategies are effective (adaptive) or ineffective (maladaptive).
    - Effective strategies control anxiety and lead to problem solving.
    - Ineffective strategies can lead to abuse of food, tobacco, drugs, or alcohol (see Classification of Coping Strategies at the end of this tab).
- **Stress tolerance:** The capacity to manage threats to self-integrity.

The focus of the coping–stress tolerance pattern is on:

- Individual, family, and community coping strategies.
- Effectiveness of strategies.
- Use of stress prevention health practices.

Why This Pattern Is Important

The following are reasons that individuals, families, and communities require assessment of this pattern:

- Coping has to occur in the patient's transition from self-as-healthy to self-as-ill or self-as-chronically-ill. Successful coping results in healthy disease management.

- Perception of an event, situation, object, or relationship as stressful is individual. Assuming that an event is or is not stressful can result in error. Perception is influenced by culture, values, and past experience.
- Denial during the acute phase of a serious illness, such as myocardial infarction, is usually a beneficial coping strategy. Time is necessary to integrate the threatening event. Denial that continues after the acute phase can be detrimental. It interferes with rehabilitation.
- Assessment of coping strategies prior to major surgery will identify patients at high risk for perioperative anxiety.
- Events that strain coping capacities, such as war, murder, major accidents, community disasters, rape, or violence, can result in post-trauma syndrome.
- Individuals can develop chronic problems over many years if post-trauma syndrome is not diagnosed and treated. If the trauma or disaster is widespread, whole communities can be affected.
- Assessment of a traumatic event's severity will provide an indicator of need for early intervention and treatment.
- Families and communities need to have a plan in place for emergency management of such necessities as communications, medicine, housing, water, and food.
- Support systems, such as a network of friends and family, are an important factor in coping with stressors.
- Self-mutilation, as a means of reducing tension, is a strategy used by a small percentage ($<1\%$) of young women. The percentage of young men using this coping strategy is unclear but less than that of women.
- Job stress is common in many workplaces. Similar to other types of stress, sustained autonomic arousal can lead to (Welker-Hood, 2006):
  - Hypertension.
  - Cardiovascular diseases.
  - Musculoskeletal disorders.
  - Impaired immunity.
  - Depression.
  - Suicide.

Individual Assessment

It is difficult to estimate the amount of stress that a particular threatening event will cause a person. It is the person's appraisal of the stressor and its meaning that influence the impact the stressor will have. Stress in life is inevitable; thus, individuals need to learn effective coping strategies. The focus of individual assessment is on:

- Stressors and stress tolerance.
- Coping patterns and their effectiveness.

Individuals at Risk

Some individuals are at increased risk for problems in this area. Be sensitive to cues when assessing individuals with any of the following characteristics:

- Uncertainty in diagnosis or prognosis.
- Financial problems.
- Marital problems.
- Interpersonal conflict.
- Health-related decisional conflict.
- Poor job fit.
- High demand/low control jobs.
- High job effort/low reward.
- Few close friends and family.

Assessment Items

History
- Have someone helpful in talking things over? That person available to you now?
- Tense or relaxed most of the time? What helps?
- Use medicines, drugs, or alcohol to relax?
- Big changes in your life in the last year or two?
- When problems occur, how do you handle them? Most of the time, is this way successful?

Examination
- Anxiety on a scale from 1 to 10, with 1 being relaxed and 10 being nervous.
- Difficulty concentrating during interview.
- Voice quivering.
- Heart rate.
- Blood pressure.

Diagnostic Categories

The following nursing diagnoses from the NANDA International Taxonomy II (2007) describe diagnostic judgments. Blue type indicates diagnoses developed by the author, not yet reviewed by NANDA, but found useful in clinical practice (Gordon, 2006).

- **Stress Overload:** Excessive amounts and types of demands that require action.
- **Ineffective Coping (Specify):** Impairment of adaptive behaviors, such as valid appraisal, choice of response, and inability to use resources. Methods of handling stressful life situations are insufficient to prevent or

control anxiety, fear, or anger. Specify stressors, such as situational or maturational crisis and uncertainty.

- **Readiness for Enhanced Coping:** Pattern of cognitive and behavioral efforts to manage demands that is sufficient for well-being and can be strengthened.
- **Avoidance Coping:** Prolonged minimization or denial of information, including facts, meanings, and consequences, when a situation requires active coping.
- **Defensive Coping:** Repeated projections of falsely positive self-evaluation based on a self-protective pattern that defends against underlying perceived threats to positive self-regard.
- **Ineffective Denial or Denial:** Conscious or unconscious attempt to reduce anxiety or fear by disavowing the knowledge or meaning of an event to the detriment of health.
- **Risk for Suicide:** Presence of risk factors for self-inflicted, life-threatening injury.
- **Support System Deficit:** Insufficient emotional or instrumental help from others.
- **Post-Trauma Syndrome:** Sustained maladaptive response to a traumatic overwhelming event.
- **Risk for Post-Trauma Syndrome:** Risk for sustained maladaptive response to a traumatic overwhelming event.
- **Self-Mutilation:** Deliberate self-injurious behavior causing tissue damage with the intent of causing nonfatal injury to attain relief of tension.
- **Risk for Self-Mutilation:** Presence of risk factors for deliberate self-injurious behavior causing tissue damage with the intent of causing nonfatal injury to attain relief of tension.

Family Assessment

Some families mobilize human and material resources and are able to withstand stressors when illness or disability occurs. Others, usually because of living with continued stress, use coping strategies that are ineffective. Coping with stressors of an illness or disability may require:

- Role-relationship changes within the family.
- Formerly dependent members assuming caregiving roles.
- Calling upon social network and community resources for assistance.

The focus of family assessment is on:

- Current stressors on family function.
- Coping strategies.
- Effectiveness of coping strategies.

Families at Risk

Some families are at increased risk for problems in this area. Be sensitive to cues when assessing families with the following characteristics:

- Lack of time for interaction or communication.
- Financial problems.
- Multiple stressors within a short period.
- Overwhelming responsibilities, such as those found in one-parent households.
- Unresolved needs, such as food, clothes, and housing.
- Less than adequate housing.
- Illness or disability of a member.

Assessment Items

History
- Big changes or difficult situations within the family in last few years? If changes: How members adapted to change?
- Family tense or relaxed most of time? If tense, what helps?
- Anyone use medicines, drugs, or alcohol to decrease tension?
- When everyday family problems arise, how handled? Most of the time, is this way successful?
- Family plans for communicating and managing emergencies?

Examination
None.

Diagnostic Categories

The following nursing diagnoses from the NANDA International Taxonomy II (2007) describe diagnostic judgments.

- **Compromised Family Coping:** Usually supportive primary person, such as a family member or close friend, providing insufficient, ineffective, or compromised support, comfort, assistance, or encouragement, which may be needed by client to manage or master adaptive tasks related to health challenge.
- **Disabled Family Coping:** Behavior of significant person, such as family member or primary person, disables own capacities and patient's capacities to effectively address tasks essential to either person's adaptation to the health challenge.
- **Readiness for Enhanced Family Coping:** Effective management of adaptive tasks involved with the patient's health challenge by family member, who now exhibits desire and readiness for enhanced health and growth in regard to self and in relation to the patient.

Community Assessment

Communities, through government departments, have a responsibility to have a plan for the occurrence of a crisis or disaster. The plan for dealing with community-wide stressors would be specific to the possible risk for the geographic area. For example:

- Tornadoes.
- Hurricanes.
- Coal mine disasters.
- Large industrial accidents.
- Terrorist attacks.
- Volatile demonstrations.

Community coping involves mobilizing government departments, people, and materials to deal with a crisis. Like individuals, communities can use ineffective coping strategies:

- Denying or minimizing the possibility of the event.
- Inadequate problem solving and planning for emergencies, such as lack of staff disaster training and evacuation planning.
- Delay in mobilization of resources.

The history of previous crises and disasters provides information to predict how a community may handle a future crisis.

Communities at Risk

Some communities are at increased risk for problems in coping with stressors. Be sensitive to cues when assessing communities with any of the following characteristics:

- Political conflicts interfering with medical disaster planning.
- Inadequate financial resources.
- Inadequate training of health-care providers for emergency management.
- Community feelings of powerlessness.
- Inadequate emergency medical systems, including police and fire services.
- High crime statistics.
- Lack of respect for personal property.
- Inadequate communication infrastructure for handling major community stressors.

Assessment Items

History (Community Representatives)

- Recent community stress? How handled?
- Current groups under stress or exhibiting tension?

- If needed: Availability of phone help lines to report need for fire, police, or medical assistance? Suicide help line?
- Groups, health-related or otherwise, trained to handle emergencies?
- Hospitals have disaster plans?

Examination
- Statistics on social problems, such as delinquency, drug abuse, alcoholism, suicide, and psychiatric illness, as measures of social stress.
- Teenage after-school recreation areas.
- Unemployment rate by race, ethnicity, and sex.
- Emergency and disaster plans.
- Designation of shelters and medical supplies (if needed for weather-related or other crisis).

Diagnostic Categories

The following nursing diagnoses from the NANDA International Taxonomy II (2007) describe diagnostic judgments.

- **Ineffective Community Coping:** Pattern of community activities for problem solving that is unsatisfactory for meeting the demands or needs of the community.
- **Readiness for Enhanced Community Coping:** Pattern of community activities for adaptation and problem solving that is satisfactory for meeting the demands or needs of the community but can be improved for management of current and future problems or stressors.

Tips for Assessing This Pattern

- Assess two important factors when a person or family is dealing with illness, disability, or other stressful event: self-esteem and a belief in the ability to cope.
- Generally, the most healthy and successful coping strategy is problem solving.
- When stress tolerance is exceeded by excessive demands that require action, stress overload occurs. Have the patient rate his or her stress level on a scale of 1 to 10. A score of 7 or above is a diagnostic cue for stress overload.
- Use probing questions to identify the cause or meaning of the stressor. The stressor has to be clear in order for an individual, family, or community to deal with the issue or problem. A statement such as "I'm always stressed out" is unclear.

- Avoid superficial assessment and premature closure on a judgment of *ineffective coping* when assessing a patient who is not managing his or her disease, medication, or dietary or activity prescription.
- Assess coping strategies during the time lapse between tests and diagnostic results, especially if traumatic news is likely.

In-Depth Assessment Tool

Classification of Coping Strategies

Coping strategies are protective psychological processes usually beyond immediate awareness. All but the first, problem solving, become unhealthy when used continuously in many areas of life or when they interfere with function (also called *defense mechanisms*). All are used at times to manage the anxiety of ineffective coping.

Coping Strategy	Description
Problem solving	Using realistic appraisal, plans, and actions to deal with a stressor and associated emotional reaction.
Compensation	Excelling in one area to overcome a real or imagined deficit in own behavior.
Rationalization	Using an excuse to justify behavior.
Denial	Not acknowledging anything that might cause emotional distress.
Repression	Placing traumatic events out of awareness so they cannot be unconsciously remembered.
Identification	Modeling oneself after the behavior or appearance of another person.
Intellectualization	Denying feelings by responding with impersonal or theoretical statements.
Regression	Behavior that is more appropriate for an earlier developmental period.
Depersonalization	Losing self-identity.
Sublimation	Redirecting an unacceptable tendency to a more acceptable one.
Suppression	Deciding consciously not to act.
Displacement	Shifting feelings from a less socially acceptable or threatening object or person to one more acceptable.

Value-Belief Pattern

The value-belief pattern describes important characteristics of individuals, families, and communities that influence health-care delivery. Two are:

- Ideals and behaviors that are important to the individual, family, or community.
- Beliefs that guide decisions and provide strength and comfort.

It is common for spirituality and values to be influenced by religious faith or belief. The socially desired outcome is morality, or moral behavior. Interrelationships among values, beliefs, and behavior are evident in the following definitions:

- **Belief** is something that is accepted as true with an emotional or spiritual sense of certainty.
- **Value** is an accepted principle or standard of an individual or group.
- **Spirituality** is a way of living that comes from a set of meanings, values, and beliefs that are important to the person. Meanings can focus on purpose in life, hope, and suffering.
- **Morality** is the practice of behavior that furthers the common good and is based in philosophical and theological principles. It is commonly referred to as good conduct.
- **Religion** is the belief in a supernatural power that has created the universe and has involvement in human life. Each religion has a set of practices, beliefs, and a theology.
- **Faith** is an inner knowing about ideas, people, and events.

The relationship between prayer and healing has roots in ancient history. Current studies suggest that a high percentage of people use prayer to prevent and cope with illness, although few people mention their use of prayer to care providers.

The Joint Commission on the Accreditation of Healthcare Organizations, the accrediting body for hospitals and other health-care agencies, requires that information be collected about spiritual needs (2000).

Why This Pattern Is Important

The following are reasons that individuals, families, and communities require assessment of this pattern:

- Beliefs and values influence decisions, goals, and actions. Knowing those related to health may provide reasons the nurse can use to motivate improved disease and health management.
- Knowing the wishes of a person or person's family provides information if an ethical issue arises, such as surgery, treatments, or the need to use advance directives.

VALUE/
BELIEF

VALUE/ BELIEF

- Privacy of medical information is a value held by patients. It is derived from the ethical principle of autonomy (Grace, 2004).
- Studies reveal that nearly two-thirds of Americans say religion is very important in their lives, 19 of 20 people say they believe in God.
- Individual practices may differ from book descriptions due to diversity among and within religions in the United States.
- Many individuals and families use prayer as a coping strategy during illness and crises.
- Spiritual values may be of even greater importance in care when an illness is prolonged, progressive, or life-threatening.
- Knowing the religion of a patient or family and their wishes regarding hospital chaplain visits can be used to assist them to meet a spiritual need.
- With no pathophysiology to justify the death, some people who are hopeless and despairing (spiritual distress) are more likely to die or die sooner than would be expected. (Harkreader and Hogan, 2004, p. 1194). Without hope, there appears to be no will to live.

Individual Assessment

Values and beliefs, including religious affiliations, can influence health beliefs. In turn, health beliefs can affect:

- Ideas about cause of an illness.
- Dietary patterns.
- Treatment options.
- Postmortem care.

The focus of individual assessment of this pattern is on:

- Important values.
- Plans for the future.
- Spiritual or religious affiliation.
- Spiritual support and religious needs.

Individuals at Risk

Some individuals are at increased risk for problems in this area. Be sensitive to cues when assessing individuals with any of the following characteristics:

- Life transitions, such as maturational transitions and retirement.
- Cultural barrier to practicing religion.
- Terminal illness.
- Uncontrolled pain or chronic pain.
- Loss of significant person, pet, job, body part, or bodily function.

- Decisional conflict, such as choice between equally risky alternatives.
- Values conflict.
- Lack of social support.
- Loneliness.

History
- Generally get things you want out of life? Most important things in your life?
- If appropriate: Plans for the future?
- Religion important in your life? If yes: Does this help when difficulties arise? Will being here interfere with any religious practices? See the Jarel Spiritual Well-Being Scale below for in-depth assessment.

As you are concluding the history or following the examination, ask the following:

- For the patient who is hospitalized: Things that are important to you while you are here? Maybe things we did not discuss?
- For the patient at a clinic visit: Things important to you at this visit that we did not discuss?

Examination
- Notice signs of worship, such as a rosary, shawl, cross, or religious pictures.

The following nursing diagnoses from the NANDA International Taxonomy II (2007) describe diagnostic judgments in this area.

- **Moral Distress:** Response to the inability to carry out one's chosen ethical or moral decision or action.
- **Spiritual Distress:** Impaired ability to experience and integrate meaning and purpose in life through connectedness with self, others, art, music, literature, or a power greater than oneself.
- **Risk for Spiritual Distress:** Presence of risk factors for an impaired ability to experience and integrate meaning and purpose in life through a connectedness with self, others, art, music, literature, nature, and/or a power greater than oneself.
- **Readiness for Enhanced Spiritual Well-Being:** Ability to experience and integrate meaning and purpose in life through connectedness with self, others, art, music, literature, nature, and/or a power greater than oneself.

VALUE/
BELIEF

- **Impaired Religiosity:** Impaired ability to rely on beliefs or participate in rituals of a particular faith tradition.
- **Risk for Impaired Religiosity:** Presence of risk factors for impaired ability to rely on religious beliefs or participate in rituals of a particular faith tradition.
- **Readiness for Enhanced Religiosity:** Desire and ability to increase reliance on religious beliefs or participate in rituals of a particular faith community.

Family Assessment

Family assessment focuses on family values and beliefs that are health-related. These include:

- Responsibility for passing on to children:
  - Cultural and moral values.
  - Spiritual values and beliefs.
- Family traditions.
- Meaning and value of relationships.
- Interconnectedness of family members.
- Meaning of family life.
- Spiritual values that can give hope and comfort during:
  - Family maturational transitions or crises.
  - Physiological or psychological crises.
  - Situational crises.

Families at Risk

Some families are at increased risk for problems in this area. Be sensitive to cues when assessing families with any of the following characteristics:

- Single-parent family without extended family support.
- Recent death of a family member.
- Drug or alcohol abuse issues.
- Poor family and neighborhood role models.
- Recent retirement of family member.
- Social rejection or alienation.
- Terminally ill family member.
- Suffering of family member.
- Family member with depression.

Assessment Items

History
- Family generally gets things it wants out of life?
- Important things for the future?
- Family rules about behavior that everyone believes are important?
- Religion important in family? If yes: Does religion help when difficulties arise?

Examination
- Notice signs of worship, such as rosary, shawl, cross, or religious pictures.

Diagnostic Categories

No family diagnoses have been identified in this pattern.

Community Assessment

Ideally, communities support the values of the families residing in the community by:
- Providing spiritual support through parks, flowers, and concerts on the green.
- Providing opportunities for people to get to know each other and serve as support systems for each other when necessary.
- Supporting businesses that serve needs and support moral values of the residents.
- Facilitating the development of churches, synagogues, temples, and mosques to meet the religious needs of residents.

Communities at Risk

Some communities are at increased risk for problems in this area. Be sensitive to cues when assessing communities with any of the following characteristics:
- Conflict over adult bookstores and lounges.
- Lack of concern for community aesthetics, such as flower gardens and clean streets.
- Lack of support for libraries, museums, and other cultural resources.
- Discriminatory practices.
- Lack of support for clubs, churches, and other community organizations.

VALUE/
BELIEF

Assessment Items

History (Community Representatives)

- Top four things that people living in the community see as important in their lives? (Note the health-related values and priorities.)
- Community members tend to get involved in causes or local fund-raising campaigns? (Note if any are health-related.)
- Religious groups found within the community? Places to worship available?
- People tend to tolerate differences? Tolerate behaviors not usually well accepted?

Examination

- Zoning and conservation laws.
- Community government health committee reports, including goals and priorities.
- Health budget relative to total budget.
- Parks, museums, and programs for the public.

Diagnostic Categories

No community diagnoses have been identified in this pattern.

Tips for Assessing This Pattern

- Avoid cultural or religious stereotyping of spiritual needs. Assumptions, rather than assessment, can lead to errors because individual differences exist within cultures and religions.
- Assessing spiritual needs requires concern, empathy, sensitivity, listening, and time. Listening can be, simultaneously, both diagnostic and therapeutic.
- Continued nursing assessment of a patient's need is required even after referring the need to another health team member, such as a chaplain.
- Limiting assessment to religious preference may miss individuals and families in spiritual distress, such as those patients who are searching for meaning in illness, have lost the will to live or the feeling of connectedness, and who experience feelings of abandonment when dying.
- Hospital patient records do not reflect spiritual needs assessment (Cavendish et al., 2003; Byrne, 2002; Broten, 1997).

In-Depth Assessment Tool

Jarel Spiritual Well-Being Scale

Directions: Please circle the choice that best describes how much you agree with each statement. Circle only one answer for each statement. There are no right or wrong answers or good or bad scores. The purpose of this scale is to help the patient talk about his or her spirituality in a nonthreatening way and to give you a sense of the importance of spirituality in your patient's life so that you can plan appropriate interventions.

	Strongly Agree (SA)	Moderately Agree (MA)	Agree (A)	Disagree	Moderately Disagree (MD)	Strongly Disagree (SD)
1. Prayer is an important part of my life.						
2. I believe I have spiritual well-being.						
3. As I grow older, I find myself more tolerant of others' beliefs						
4. I find meaning and purpose in my life						
5. I feel there is a close relationship between my spiritual beliefs and what I do.						
6. I believe in an afterlife.						
7. When I am sick, I have less spiritual well-being.						

VALUE/ BELIEF

Jarel Spiritual Well-Being Scale

	Strongly Agree (SA)	Moderately Agree (MA)	Agree (A)	Disagree	Moderately Disagree (MD)	Strongly Disagree (SD)
8. I believe in a Supreme Power.						
9. I am able to receive love from and give love to others.						
10. I am satisfied with my life.						
11. I set goals for myself.						
12. God has little meaning in my life.						
13. I am satisfied with the way I am using my abilities.						
14. Prayer does not help me in making decisions.						
15. I am able to appreciate differences in others.						
16. I am pretty well put together.						
17. I prefer that others make decisions for me.						
18. I find it hard to forgive others.						

Jarel Spiritual Well-Being Scale

	Strongly Agree (SA)	Moderately Agree (MA)	Agree (A)	Disagree	Moderately Disagree (MD)	Strongly Disagree (SD)
19. I accept my life situations.						
20. Belief in a Supreme Being has no part in my life.						
21. I cannot accept changes in my life.						

Adapted from Hungelmann J, Kenkel-Rossi E, Klassen L, and Stollenwerk, R (1987). Marquette University College of Nursing, Milwaukee, Wisconsin.

VALUE/ BELIEF

Assessment Data: Analysis and Interpretation

The purpose of gathering assessment data is to evaluate the health status of an individual, family, or community. This evaluation is based on an analysis and interpretation of the assessment data.

Analysis and interpretation of data require cognitive judgment skills and a vocabulary to communicate the judgments:

- The diagnostic process describes the reasoning skills used in clinical judgment.
- The NANDA International Taxonomy II provides a nursing diagnosis vocabulary for recording and communicating diagnostic judgments (NANDA-I, 2007). Taxonomy is a systematic arrangement of diagnosis within a category system.

Diagnosis Vocabulary

A diagnosis is specified as a nursing diagnosis when it is necessary to distinguish a diagnosis made by a nurse from that of a physician or other health-care professional. Identifying and standardizing nursing diagnoses are the focus of various groups around the world.

- The International Council of Nurses is developing an International Classification for Nursing Practice (ICNP) that includes diagnoses and interventions (see www.icn.ch/icnp.htm).
- Various languages within the United States have also developed a language for practice. NANDA International is the most representative group and has been developing diagnoses since 1973 (see Tab 15 for current diagnoses).

Diagnostic Categories for Summarizing Assessment Data

Diagnostic categories, or nursing diagnoses, summarize the assessment data into meaningful clusters of information. They are a shorthand way of describing a health state. The following are characteristics of nursing diagnoses:

- State a problem, a risk state, or a readiness for a higher-level wellness.
- Have a concept with a name, definition, specific defining characteristics (signs and symptoms), and etiological or related factors.
- Belong to a class or category in a diagnostic classification system, such as the NANDA International Taxonomy II.
- Describe a condition of an individual, family, or community, resolved primarily through nursing intervention.
- Made by a professional nurse (Nurse Practice Act).
- Allow communication of what nurses do and is a building block of nursing science.

A nursing diagnosis is not to be confused with the following:

■ Not a nursing treatment, such as emotional support.
■ Not a medical diagnosis, such as congestive heart failure.
■ Not a tube, such as a Foley catheter.
■ Not individual signs or symptoms, such as angry or crying.
■ Not a procedure, such as suctioning.
■ Not a patient need, such as teaching.

Components of a Clinically Useful Nursing Diagnosis

■ **Name:** Clear and concise standardized label.
■ **Definition:** Summarization of the characteristics of the condition.
■ **Defining characteristics:** Diagnostic and supporting cues.
■ **Etiology or related factors:** Probable reasons for the condition.
■ **High-risk groups:** People who are at increased risk for the condition (Gordon, 2007). (This last component not used by NANDA International.)

PES Format

A diagnostic statement contains the problem and etiology but is documented with the supporting signs and symptoms. This is referred to as the PES format:

■ **Problem:** Diagnosis name that describes the state of the patient.
■ **Etiology or related factors:** Describes the probable cause(s) of the problem.
■ **Signs and symptoms:** Data that support the problem and etiology.

Definition of Nursing Diagnosis

The definition of nursing diagnosis used by NANDA International communicates important ideas about contemporary professional nursing practice, vocabulary, and the use of diagnosis within the nursing process. The definition approved in 1990 is: "A nursing diagnosis is a clinical judgment about an individual, family, or community response to actual or potential health problems or life processes. A nursing diagnosis provides the basis for selection of nursing interventions to achieve outcomes for which the nurse is accountable" (NANDA-I, 2007).

The ideas captured in the definition have influenced contemporary practice and standards of care (Tab 1):

■ Nurses make diagnostic judgments.
■ Nursing interventions are specific to the nursing diagnosis.
■ The nurse is accountable for achieving outcomes related to the nursing diagnosis.

Diagnostic Process

The diagnostic process consists of cue recognition, strategies for information interpretation, and the final judgment about a nursing diagnosis. It takes many words to describe the diagnostic reasoning process, but a working diagnosis usually happens within a minute as the experienced nurse is assessing.

Cue Recognition

The diagnostic process begins with the first cue obtained during assessment of a health pattern and the need to explain its occurrence. *Cue* refers to a sign or symptom. A diagnostic cue is a sign or symptom that has to be present to make the diagnosis. Diagnostic cues are the criteria for nursing diagnosis. Accuracy in cue recognition is a critically important component of assessment. It affects everything from diagnosis to care delivery. Because of their importance, consider the factors that may affect cue recognition:

- **Clinical knowledge** relevant to the practice area.
- **Organization of clinical knowledge** in memory for easy retrieval when needed during interpretation of assessment data.
- **Selective attention** to assessment with no distractions or interruptions.
- **Clarity of scope of practice** and knowing what information is important.
- **Curiosity** to wonder why, when encountering the unusual or unexpected.
- **Fatigue** that may decrease sensitivity to cues.

A diagnostic cue causes a shift into the diagnostic process. In contrast, if information indicates healthy behaviors, assessment continues and there is no shift toward the diagnostic process.

Diagnostic Strategies

Thinking processes within the diagnostic process can be hard to understand because they cannot be seen, heard, or touched. The idea of strategies is a useful way of describing the behavior observed when a nurse is reasoning from data to diagnosis. Strategies, which are usually not conscious, have the following characteristics:

- Used to acquire, combine, integrate, and interpret the meaning of data to make a diagnosis.
- Described as analytic reasoning and intuition. The former employs inductive and deductive inference.
- Observed to differ between experts and novices.

Analytic Reasoning Strategies

The inexperienced novice as well as the expert encountering an unfamiliar clinical problem use analytic strategies. These strategies are also useful in complex, diagnostic tasks in which there is no prior experience with the condition. Features of analytic strategy are the following:

- Defined as logical, critical, or rational thinking.
- Uses divergent thinking to generate alternative explanations for a cue and convergent thinking to focus cue search. See the figure below depicting generation of multiple hypotheses to explain the cues as branches on a tree. Going down one branch to check one hypothesis requires convergent thinking.

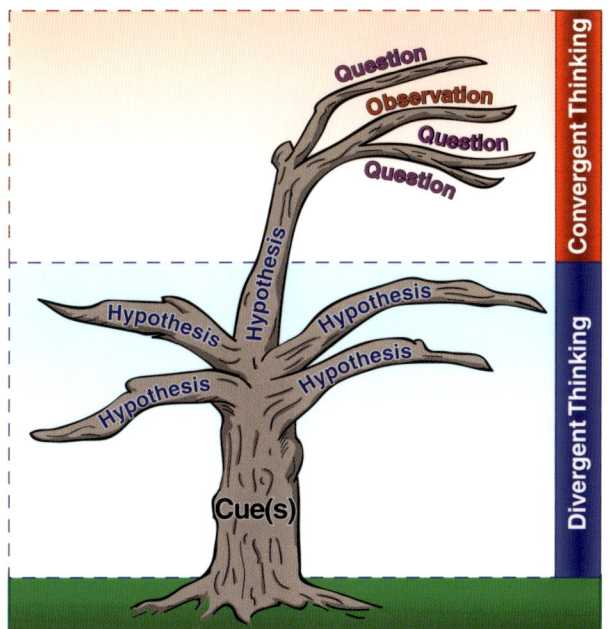

- Uses step-by-step reasoning and rules for combining data for diagnosis.
- Facilitated by knowledge organized in memory for easy retrieval as needed during assessment
- Requires validation of diagnostic judgments.

Diagnostic Strategies: Intuition

Intuitive inference is defined as immediate insight without conscious deliberation or analysis. Expert nurses with many years of experience in a specific area frequently use intuition in problem identification but can use analytic strategies when indicated. Features of intuition are the following:

- Recognize similarities in situations, and use past experiences for interpretation.
- Use previous patients as reference points for recognizing the cue pattern of a diagnosis, similar to case-based reasoning.
- Developed through a combination of thinking, doing, and reflecting on practice.
- Requires validation of intuitions when possible.

Interpretation of Data Using Analytic Strategies

Analysis and interpretation of the data using an analytic strategy involve generating possible hypotheses, searching for their diagnostic criteria, and a judgment about which possibility is supported.

Hypothesis Generation

Recognizing a cue, such as verbal report of fatigue, causes possible hypotheses, or interpretations, to come to mind. These hypotheses are useful in thinking because they provide:

- Possible explanations of the cues.
- Diagnostic criteria that directly search for cues.
- Focus for further assessment that will be the basis for a diagnostic judgment.

Hypotheses may be at different levels. They may be broad problems, such as a nutritional problem, or specific nursing diagnoses, such as nutritional deficit. This depends on the information available during assessment when a cue is initially recognized. The generation of hypotheses from clinical knowledge and current assessment information:

Requires divergent thinking to generate hypotheses as depicted in the earlier figure. Patient report of tiredness or fatigue, for example, would generate five hypotheses, similar to five branches of a tree: nutritional deficit, sleep apnea, sleep deprivation, a cardiac or respiratory problem, and activity intolerance.

- Begins to frame the problem and provide alternative meanings. Reframing is useful when a new perspective is needed. This occurs when hypotheses are not supported. For example, if cues do not support any of the above hypotheses, then a new perspective is needed.
- Requires flexible thinking and well-organized clinical knowledge.

Alternative Hypotheses

Generate two or more alternate hypotheses. Alternative explanations increase the probability that the correct one is included. Avoid having to say, "I never thought of that!"

There are a number of sources that can be used to generate diagnostic hypotheses or possibilities. The following are examples (Gordon, 1994, 164–177):

- **Health pattern being assessed:** Using the pattern narrows down the possibilities. Example: If assessing the role-relationship pattern, use the pattern as the working hypothesis: relationship problem.
- **Diagnoses within pattern being assessed:** Cues may suggest a particular diagnosis. Review diagnoses grouped within the pattern being assessed, and use relevant diagnoses as tentative hypotheses. Try to commit the diagnoses common in your practice to memory. See Tab 15 for diagnoses grouped by each individual functional health pattern.
- **Health pattern sequence and relationships:** Information from one pattern may help explain a cue in another pattern. For example, a verbal report of being nervous (self-perception/self-concept pattern) may explain a cue of trouble sleeping (sleep-rest pattern). Sedentary activity or dietary pattern may explain a reason for the cue of weight exceeding norm.
- **Patient's viewpoint:** The patient's perspective is always important. It may also help to develop possible explanations for the data. Ask one of the following questions:
  - What do you think that means?
  - What do you think that is?
  - Why do you think that happened?

When asking these questions, use an empathetic, questioning tone to elicit information that may suggest diagnostic hypotheses for further assessment.

- **Background knowledge:** Previously learned information from textbooks, experts, and research is a common source of hypotheses.
- **Examples and generalizations from experience:** These are useful but can lead to error if assumptions are not checked against further data collection.
- **Contextual information:** Factors in the setting: age group, acuity level, medical or psychiatric diagnosis, observations of the surroundings, and ongoing treatments can be a source of tentative diagnostic hypotheses about assessment data.

- **Personal theories:** Implicit theories about prognosis, types of people, or situations can be a source of hypotheses during assessment. Be careful that personal theories do not bias judgments or lead to negative stereotyping. For example, a care provider who believes there is no future with terminal illness may interpret future-oriented planning by a terminally ill patient as denial of illness.
- **Empathy:** The nurse's own feelings are used to generate hypotheses about the feelings, acts, or behaviors of the person being assessed. Example: Patient is a young working mother, and the nurse is a young working mother. Nurse uses her understanding of role demands to anticipate possible problems of the patient. This is usually a successful strategy if similarities are shared. Hypotheses must be validated.
- **Initial impressions:** Formed early in the interaction, initial impressions can be the basis for tentative diagnostic hypotheses. Although useful, these can lead to bias and stereotyping if not validated.

The more information obtained, the less chance of incorrect hypotheses. When information is ambiguous or incomplete, people fill in the blanks with inference or assumptions. Verify and validate.

Selecting Hypotheses
After identifying multiple possibilities, determine the most likely hypotheses by considering:

- Patient, family, or community profile.
- Information about the incidence of the possible problems identified.
- Assessment information already collected.

Hypothesis Testing

Hypothesis testing is a focused and efficient search for cues to confirm or reject tentative hypotheses. When testing diagnostic hypotheses, the nurse:

- **Tests the most likely hypotheses first.**
- **Uses convergent thinking:** This is focused on testing for the presence of characteristics that have to be present to confirm a hypothesis. Focus on diagnostic cues first.
- **Uses observations and questions to test for the presence of the diagnosis:** If all diagnostic cues are present, the diagnosis is supported.
- **Discards the diagnostic hypotheses that were not supported:** This reduces the number of possible hypotheses.

When it is not possible to make a diagnosis, the usual procedure is to document "rule out" (R/O) and to continue to collect information. For example: R/O *Dysfunctional Family Processes.*

Formulating the Diagnostic Statement

During formulation of the diagnostic statement, there are a number of factors to consider. These are reviewing the database and judgments made during assessment and the structure and content of the diagnostic statement that will summarize the data.

Final Review of Database and Judgments

- The nurse makes a final review of notes taken while assessing the health patterns. Notes will be in the form of:
  - Assessment data.
  - Problems or risk states.
  - Etiological or related factors.
  - Strengths or patterns that are functional.
- A synthesis is needed after all patterns have been assessed. Think about the problems and strengths identified in the context of the whole person, family, or community that was assessed. Is there a need to revise any problems? Consider the following two examples:
  - Data may support the diagnosis of *Impaired parenting,* but the practice observed is accepted in the patient's culture. Delete or revise.
  - Data may support *Noncompliance with dietary prescription.* In a hospice setting, a nurse probably would not diagnose and treat noncompliance.
- Check that the diagnostic cues that have to be present to make an accurate diagnosis (Gordon, 2007) are present.
- Make your diagnoses as precise as possible. The more precise the diagnosis, the easier it is to develop interventions. For example:
  - *Impaired skin integrity* is too broad; specify the type of impairment.
  - *Risk for infection* is too broad for a localized infection. Use a more specific diagnosis, such as *Risk for respiratory infection* or *Risk for urinary tract infection.*
- Check that there are sufficient risk factors identified that can be reduced by *nursing* care when making a risk diagnosis.

Structure and Content of the Diagnostic Statement

The diagnostic statement consists of the problem and the etiology or related factors. Documentation includes the supporting signs and symptoms for the problem and etiology. When structuring the diagnostic statement, remember these tips:

- Describe the problem, which is the state of the patient, family, or community, as a nursing diagnosis using standard terminology (NANDA International, 2007).
- Describe the probable causes of the problem, that is, the etiological or related factors, in concise terms. Use the NANDA International Taxonomy II for terms when possible because these are defined and have defining characteristics specified.

- Structure the diagnostic statement as in the following examples: *Self-care deficit, Level 2 related to activity intolerance, Anxiety related to acute pain, Situational low self-esteem related to disturbed body image,* and *Ineffective community coping related to ineffective role performance.*
- Formulate a clear diagnostic statement because it will be used in planning patient care.
- Identify patient outcomes based on the problem. Problem resolution or progress toward resolution is the desired outcome.
- Identify interventions for actual problems based on the *etiological* or *related factors* as above. They describe the probable cause of the problem and are the focus for nursing intervention decisions.

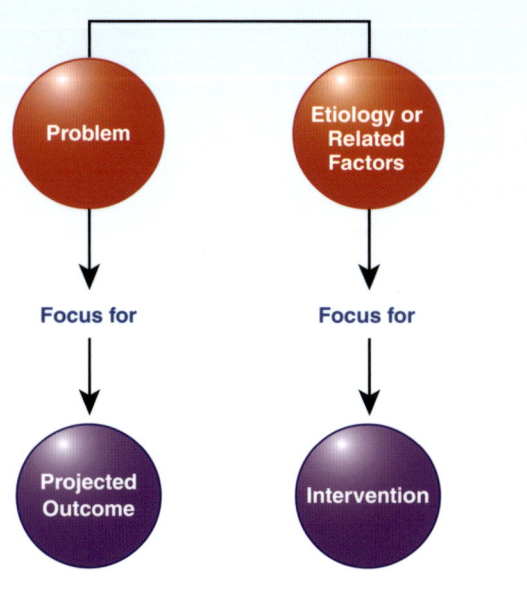

- Identify *risk diagnoses* based on a set of risk factors. The factors are used as a basis for intervention decisions. Risk reduction is the desired outcome. Risk diagnoses do not have etiological factors, as the actual problem does not exist.
- Identify *wellness diagnoses* when the patient has a functional pattern and expresses a desire to enhance; for example: *Readiness for enhanced parenting*. Etiological factors are not specified for wellness diagnoses.
- Identify strengths, that is, functional patterns, during assessment as a resource for the patient to manage problems that may be present. Functional patterns are also prerequisite to a movement toward a higher level of wellness.

Accuracy of Judgments

Accuracy in information collection and interpretation will influence intervention decisions and patient outcomes. Accuracy is enhanced by:

- Observations devoid of misperceptions and bias.
- Measurement that is accurate.
- Cue investigation that is comprehensive.
- Diagnostic interpretations that are clear and precise.
- Problem identification strongly supported by data.
- Etiological or related factors strongly supported by data and with a causal relationship to the problem that can be justified.

Sources of Error

Errors can be reduced with knowledge of diagnostic categories and their diagnostic and supporting cues. In any one clinical setting, there are probably not more than 10 diagnoses used every day. These diagnoses and their diagnostic cues are easily learned. Others can be added as less common problems are recognized. Common sources of and possible reasons for errors are:

- Information collection errors:
  - Not observing cues, which can be caused by lack of categories, distraction, or fatigue.
  - Observing but not recognizing a cue as relevant, which can be caused by lack of knowledge about the category.
  - Overload of information, which can include a lack of systematic approach to assessment.
  - Method, including less than adequate attention or technical skill in measuring a characteristic.

- Information interpretation errors:
  - Not taking individual, developmental, and cultural norms into account; lack of cultural knowledge or motivation to individualize care.
  - Overgeneralizing or limited observation.
  - Inadequately validating subjective inferences and hypotheses with the patient; not obtaining verbal reports when diagnoses are subjective states or processes.
  - Not revising hypotheses in light of new data or not reframing from another diagnostic perspective; holding onto an idea when new data say to reject.
  - Premature closure on a diagnosis; making a diagnosis before sufficient data are collected; lack of knowledge of diagnostic criteria.
- Diagnosis formulation errors:
  - Not recognizing inconsistencies in formulating a diagnostic statement. Cues contradict the identified problem.
  - Not following the "rules" for language usage.
  - Lack of knowledge of category definitions and defining characteristics.
  - Diagnosis too broad to guide intervention decisions.
  - Lack of branching questions and observations for a precise diagnosis; lack of knowledge of diagnoses in an area.
  - Etiological and related factors attributed to person's behavior, when reason lies in the situation (also the reverse); not adequately assessing alternative reasons for a condition.
  - Specifying medical diagnosis as an etiological factor, which is not a focus for nursing intervention.
  - Inadequate assessment or not using a nursing perspective to generate possible causal factors.

Common Concerns

Some common concerns about functional health pattern assessment include time, number of patterns that must be assessed, losing the focus on the medical diagnosis, and data to prevent or resolve ethical issues.

Time

Nurses are worried that this type of assessment takes too much time. Actually, the time to complete an assessment varies greatly, depending on the following factors:

- Complexity of the medical and nursing problems.
- Level of the patient's anxiety that influences the admission interview.
- Complexity of the social problems.

- Expertise of the nurse in health pattern assessment.
- Amount of explaining, teaching, and other interventions included in the admission assessment.

For an admission assessment, it is worth the time to identify risk factors and problems and establish a therapeutic relationship with the patient or, if a home visit, the family.

Number of Patterns to Assess

Nurses ask themselves whether all patterns should be assessed on admission or just those that are relevant. When asking yourself this question, remember that all patterns are relevant because you do not yet know which patterns are not relevant until they have been assessed.

Also consider that:

- Medical diagnoses are not reliable predictors of the scope of nursing diagnoses. Medical diagnoses are in the pathophysiological or psychopathological domain, and nursing diagnoses are in the biopsychosocial-spiritual domain.
- Screening questions in each pattern may suffice when it is not possible to do a full assessment. For example, "Mr. G., do you have any problems with diet, eating, or indigestion? Any problems with bowels or passing your water?"
- After a screening assessment, the registered nurse can obtain further information during care.
- A full assessment is mandated by law in long-term care settings on admission and periodically thereafter.

Losing the Focus on the Medical Diagnosis

Assessment is expanded in those patterns directly affected by the disease. For example:

- The history would be expanded in the activity-exercise pattern with a disease involving the lungs.
- Examination would include a pulmonary and chest assessment.
- The nurse will know the medical diagnosis and keep it in mind. It will be one of the variable factors taken into account in the assessment of each pattern:
  - Age.
  - Developmental level.
  - Gender.
  - Culture.
  - Medical diagnosis (if present).

Resolving Ethical Issues

During care delivery, an ethical issue may arise. In a number of cases, resolution requires the kind of information collected by nurses. For example:

- Cognitive-perceptual pattern data are useful in determining decision-making capacity and the need for a substitute decision maker.
- Health perception–health management pattern data identify patient understanding of diagnosis and treatment, a factor necessary for signing consent for treatment.
- Value-belief pattern data may be used in determining wishes about life-sustaining and other treatments.

Common Dilemmas in Data Interpretation

The following are dilemmas that nurses and students commonly encounter in the interpretation and summarization of assessment data:

- **Following an assessment, there are no diagnostic cues.** Consider that:
  - There are no health problems.
  - The assessment was superficial; cues were missed.
  - Hypotheses were not generated to guide branching questions and observations.
- **You have the cluster of cues but have no idea of the problem.** This could be caused by:
  - Insufficient knowledge of diagnoses and diagnostic cues; that is, the criteria for using categories.
  - More than one diagnosis in the cluster of cues.
- **Nothing fits the cues.** This could be caused by:
  - Insufficient or no diagnostic cues due to inadequate hypothesis generation and testing.
  - Cues signifying a disease, disease complication, or adverse effect of medical therapy. Report findings to physician.
  - Cues representing a condition within the scope of nursing that has not been named. Check how to create a nursing diagnosis (NANDA-I, 2007).
- **Many problems have been formulated.** When this happens, it may be because:
  - It is a multiproblem individual, family, or community. Prioritize according to acuity level or impact on quality of life.
  - A final synthesis of the problems identified was not done. If causal links or relationships among problems are determined in the problem-etiology format, there may be fewer problems.

- There may be a syndrome; that is, a cluster of problems with the same etiology. Diagnoses such as *Activity intolerance* or *Self-care deficit* may cause multiple problems.
- **Problem formulated may or may not be a nursing diagnosis.** When this happens, keep in mind the following:
  - A common mistaken assumption is that everything has to be tied to the medical diagnosis. For example, the following are two diagnoses that are not clinically useful: *Activity intolerance related to chronic obstructive lung disease (COPD)* or *Low self-esteem related to hysterectomy.* Etiology is the basis for nursing intervention decisions. Nurses cannot treat COPD or hysterectomy. Assess and reformulate the above statements as follows: social isolation related to activity intolerance and sexual dysfunction related to situational low self-esteem.
  - A reformulated medical diagnosis is not a nursing diagnosis. A commonly seen type of reformulation is of the form *Multiple sclerosis to alterations in neurological status.*
- **Problem formulation is vague and imprecise.** Vague and imprecise problems cause difficulties in making decisions about interventions and outcomes. When this is the case, the problem could be:
  - Insufficient assessment. The diagnosis lacks specificity.
  - The etiological factor is a component of the problem. For example: *Fear related to worry and concern* (worry and concern are diagnostic cues to fear, not probable causes); *Self-care deficit related to bathing deficit* (bathing is a dimension of self-care deficit).
  - Nonspecific diagnoses, such as "alterations in" or "impairment." These are very imprecise. Specify the type of alteration or impairment.

Using Assessment Data: A Case Study

A simple example may help to clarify the diagnostic process for summarizing assessment data. The extensive description that follows takes the nurse approximately 2 minutes or less. Consider the case of Mr. G., whom the nurse sees during his routine visit to a physician's office. The nurse notes that Mr. G.:

- Is a 45-year-old company executive.
- Has had a medical diagnosis of essential hypertension (high blood pressure) for 3 years.

Cues Recognized

- Exhausted appearance:
  - Dark circles under eyes.

- Slow gait.
- States he is tired.
- Reports trouble sleeping.

Hypotheses Generated (Possibilities)

The nurse generates the following hypotheses from the initial observations and conversation. She makes the hypotheses general in order to avoid premature closure or focusing on one specific problem too early in the assessment. The two hypotheses selected are:

- Sleep pattern disturbance.
- Cardiac problem.

A check of the physician's note reveals the following: "no cardiac abnormality, pressure elevated, his company having financial difficulties."

Hypotheses Revised

Based on the physician's note, the nurse deletes the hypothesis of cardiac problem as a cause of his symptoms. Then the nurse reviews the diagnoses in the sleep-rest pattern to think about what sleep disturbances Mr. G. might have:

- *Insomnia.*
- *Sleep deprivation.*
- *Sleep pattern reversal.*
- *Readiness for enhanced sleep.*

With these in mind and a review of the data already collected (45-year-old male company executive whose company is experiencing financial difficulty is having difficulty sleeping), the nurse thinks about the likelihood of occurrence:

- The diagnosis *Sleep pattern reversal* is reduced. This condition is more common in an elderly person who naps most of the day and workers changing shifts.
- The diagnosis *Readiness for enhanced sleep* is deleted. Generally, this diagnosis is used to promote a higher level of wellness when sleep is adequate.
- More information will clarify whether the problem is *Delayed sleep onset* as in insomnia or a prolonged problem as in *Sleep deprivation.*
- The nurse had checked the definition and defining characteristics of *Sleep deprivation.* They are more severe than those exhibited by Mr. G. The nurse recalls that *Insomnia* is the most frequently occurring sleep disturbance in adults. This hypothesis is the most probable.

Hypothesis Testing

One broad question will produce information on the probability of the two remaining hypotheses. Exploring with Mr. G. what "trouble sleeping" means will:

- Provide information to narrow the possibilities to one.
- Provide data on the actual sleep disturbance.
- Yield information on the three remaining possibilities.

The nurse begins with an open-ended question:

Nurse: "You mentioned you were having trouble sleeping. Could you tell me more about that?"

Mr. G.: "I guess I keep thinking and can't get to sleep right away. This has been going on for the last 4 weeks. I used to sleep so well."

The nurse lets the patient know she has heard his concern and uses a focused question to get specific information:

Nurse: "That must be difficult for you and not good for your hypertension. Have you noticed how long it takes to get to sleep?"

Mr. G.: "About 2 to 4 hours, and then I just get about 3 hours of sleep."

The nurse looks for the reason for the insomnia:

Nurse: "Sometimes worries or problems can keep running through your mind when you try to get to sleep. Would that be a reason for your trouble?"

Mr. G: "For the last month, I have been trying to think of a way out, and then I can't get to sleep; I am going to lose my company to bankruptcy, and there goes my job."

The nurse begins to think about stress overload as a reason for insomnia. The next response is an intervention, but it is appropriate here.

Nurse: "That certainly is a worry for you. Is there anyone who can help you manage this? Perhaps your bank?"

The nurse now has the following cues:

- 45-year-old male.
- Company executive.
- Hypertension.
- Has trouble sleeping; keeps thinking.
- Thinking focused on: "Going to lose my company to bankruptcy, and there goes my job."
- No sleep problems prior to this time.
- Delay in sleep onset for 2 to 4 hours for 4 weeks.
- Actual sleep time about 3 hours per night.
- Bankruptcy issues started 1 month ago.

Review of Database and Judgments

A check of the diagnostic manual revals that:

■ One characteristic of *Insomnia* is a 2- to 3-hour delay before falling asleep.
■ Usually, inability to fall asleep after 30 to 45 minutes of expectation that sleep will come is diagnostic of insomnia.

Sleep deprivation is deleted; he is not "without sleep," a characteristic of this diagnosis.

Another problem was identified during the assessment:

Stress overload, defined as excessive amounts and types of demands that require action.

This diagnostic hypothesis was based on the following:

■ "For the last month, I have been trying to think of a way out, and then I can't get to sleep."
■ "I am going to lose my company to bankruptcy, and there goes my job."
■ "I keep thinking and can't get to sleep right away."
■ 45-year-old company executive and owner

Structure and Content of the Diagnostic Statement

The nurse identified two problems, *Insomnia* and *Stress overload.* Using theoretical knowledge, the nurse made the judgment that *Stress overload* was the reason for the *Insomnia.* The diagnostic statement is:

■ *Insomnia related to stress overload.* This is supported by the signs and symptoms outlined above.

Using the Diagnostic Statement

Combining the two problems in a diagnostic statement provides a basis for:

■ Outcome projection (based on *Insomnia*).
■ Intervention planning (based on *Stress overload*).

Case Study Review

The nurse completed a full functional health pattern assessment with the following in mind:

■ A careful reassessment of the role-relationship and coping-stress tolerance pattern to assess Mr. G.'s support system and coping effectiveness.
■ The patterns important in his management of essential hypertension and prevention of future complications.
■ The interaction of the nursing and medical diagnoses *Stress overload* and *Hypertension.*

Individual Assessment Guidelines*

Use the item's content to individualize questions. Keep in mind the four threads that influence every pattern and data interpretation: Culture, Age/developmental level, Disease (if present), and Sex/gender (CADS). (See Diagnostic Categories Grouped by Functional Health Patterns, 2006–2008, pp. 175–181.)

History

Health Perception–Health Management Pattern

How has your general health been?

_____

Most important things done to keep healthy?

_____

Allergies?

_____

If person has an illness: What action did you take when you perceived symptoms? Did it help?

_____

Cause of illness?

_____

Medications currently taking? Names? Dose? Times? (See Tab 3 for in-depth assessment.)

_____

Problems obtaining or taking medications? (See Tab 3 for in-depth assessment.)

_____

Medications seem to be helping?

_____

Did you bring your medications with you?

_____

Do you use any herbs or other family remedies?

_____

*See family or community assessment guidelines to clarify influencing factors.

Any colds in the past year? If so, how many?

Absences from work/school lasting longer than 1 week?
Number? Reasons?

Monthly breast self-examination? Mammogram? Prostate screening? Bone density? Colonoscopy? Pap smear? (Circle if Yes.)
If in high-risk group: Flu and pneumonia vaccinations? Tetanus booster? Hepatitis vaccination? Other age-appropriate immunizations? (Circle if Yes.)
Use cigarettes? Drugs? Alcohol? (Circle if Yes.)
Any accidents (home, work, driving)? (Circle if Yes.)
Falls in the past year?

In the past, has it been easy to follow suggestions/recommendations of doctors or nurses? (If the patient is ineffectively managing his or her health, see Tab 3 for in-depth assessment.)

If appropriate: What things are important to you while you are here?

How can we be helpful?

Nutritional-Metabolic Pattern
Typical daily food intake?

Supplements? _____ Vitamins? _____
Type and timing of snacks?

Weight: _____ lb Circle one: Stable/Loss/Gain
Height: _____ Loss? _____ Amount: _____ in
Appetite?

Food or eating discomfort? Problems swallowing?

Diet restrictions?

Able to follow restrictions?

If appropriate: Breastfeeding?

Typical daily fluid intake. Describe.

Heal well or poorly?

Skin problems: Lesions? Dryness?

Dry mouth?

Dental problems? Bleeding gums?

Elimination Pattern
Bowel elimination pattern?

Frequency? _____ Character? _____ Discomfort? _____
Problem in control?

Lose bowel contents when do not want to?

Describe bowel continence.

Use of laxatives? _____ Other methods _____
Urinary elimination pattern?

Frequency?

Trouble holding your urine (water) until get to bathroom?

Lose urine when do not want to (e.g., sneezing, coughing,
laughing)? _____ If yes: wear a pad? _____
Interfere with your activities?

Excess perspiration? _____
Odor problems? _____
Body cavity drainage (e.g., catheter, ostomy), suction, etc.?
_____

Activity-Exercise Pattern (See In-Depth Assessment tools in Tab 5, Elimination)
Sufficient energy for desired or required activities (e.g., work/school/home)?
_____

Describe activity level for most days of the week:
Very active _____
Moderately active _____
Sedentary _____
Exercise pattern? _____

Type?
_____
_____

Regularity?
_____

Hours/week?
_____

Spare time (leisure activities):
Type? _____
Alone or with others? _____
In last few months: Unsteady gait? _____ Dizziness? _____
Fainting? _____ Falls? _____
Person's perceived ability for activities of daily living (Code 1–4 according to Functional Levels Code below):

Feeding _____	Grooming _____
Bathing _____	General mobility _____
Toileting _____	Cooking _____
Bed mobility _____	Home maintenance _____
Dressing _____	Shopping _____

Functional Levels Code (From NANDA International, 2005)
0: Independent.
1: Requires use of equipment or device.
2: Requires assistance or supervision of another person.
3: Requires assistance or supervision of another person and equipment or device.
4: Is dependent and does not participate.

Sleep-Rest Pattern
Generally feel rested and ready for daily activities after sleep?

(If sleep problem, see Tab 7 for in-depth assessment.)
Sleep onset problems?
Aids to sleep used?
(If sleep problem, see Tab 7 for in-depth assessment.)
Dreams/night awakenings?

Snoring?

Headache when awakening?

Ever doze off for a second when driving?

Rest/relaxation periods during day?

Cognitive-Perceptual Pattern
Any discomfort or pain?

(If present, see Tab 8 for in-depth assessment.)
Location?

When occurs?

Associated with?

When pain first started?

Quality?

What seems to help when pain occurs?

Effective most of the time?

Any difficulty in vision?

Wear glasses? _____ Date last checked? _____
Use contact lens? _____

Difficulty hearing? _____

If yes: Hearing aid? _____
Use aid frequently? _____
Exposed to loud noise/music? _____

Any changes in taste of food? _____

Change in sense of smell? _____

Any changes in feeling/touch of toes, feet, hands? _____

Any change in memory? _____
If yes, recent things? _____
Things from the past? _____
If yes: How interferes with activities? _____

Today's date? _____ Day of week? _____
Current President of U.S.? _____
Name of this place? _____
Any problems in concentration? _____
If yes: Feel this interferes with tasks/work? _____

Are decisions easy or difficult to make? _____

If difficult: describe the difficulty: _____

(If impaired decision making is suspected, grade using the Judgment and
Decision-Making Scale in Tab 8.)

Any difficulty learning? _____

Ever told you have learning disability? _____

Easiest way you learn? What helps?

Level of school completed?

Self-Perception–Self-Concept Pattern
How would you describe yourself?

Most of the time, feel good (not so good) about yourself?

Changes in your body or the things you can do? Are these a problem for you?

Changes in way you feel about yourself or your body (since illness started)?

Find things frequently make you angry? _____
Annoyed? _____ Fearful? _____ Anxious? _____ Depressed? _____
What helps when this happens?

(If indicated, see Risk Factors for Depression in Elderly in Tab 9.)
Ever feel you lose hope?

Ever feel you are not able to control things in life?

What helps?

(If appropriate and there are concerns about death, see Assessing Fears About Death in Tab 9.)

Role-Relationship Pattern
Live alone? _____
Family structure (diagram)? _____
Any family problems difficult to handle (nuclear/extended family)?

How are problems usually handled?

Family or others depend on you for things?
_____

If hospital admission or emergency room: How are they managing now?
_____
_____

(If caregiver role strain suspected, see Caregiving Needs Checklist, Tab 10.)
Any recent losses; someone close to you?
_____

If appropriate: How family/others are responding to your
illness/hospitalization?
_____

If appropriate: Problems with children?
_____

Any difficulty handling these problems?
_____

If appropriate and if married or living with partner: How do you and your
husband/partner settle arguments?
_____

Do you feel safe in your current relationship?
_____

(This item is designed to screen for domestic violence [men and women].
Some health-care facilities require this screening. It is recommended that
assessment include this question and that it be administered without the
partner present. See Tab 10, Screening for Domestic Violence, for in-depth
assessment.)
Belong to social groups (veterans, rotary, golf club, church groups, etc.)?
_____

Close friend with whom you confide?
_____

Ever feel lonely (if yes, how often)?
_____

Things generally go well at work?
_____

School? _____
If appropriate: Income sufficient for needs?
_____
_____

Feel part of (or isolated from) neighborhood where you are living?

_____

Sexuality-Reproductive Pattern
Female: When menstruation started? _____

Last menstrual period? _____
Any problems? _____
Para? _____ Gravida? _____
If appropriate to age: Use of family planning?

Use of birth control medications? _____
Problems?

_____

If person is married: Sexual relationship in your marriage satisfying?

Any problems?

If person is unmarried: Sexually active? _____
If yes: Any problems in your sexual relations?

If person is elderly married: Any change in your and your wife's/husband's interest in sex?

Unmarried elderly: Any sexual problems?

Coping–Stress Tolerance Pattern
Have someone who is helpful in talking things over?

_____

That person available to you now?

Tense or relaxed most of the time? _____
What helps?

Use any medicines, drugs, or alcohol to relax?

Any big changes in your life in the last year or two?

_____

When big problems (or any problems) occur in your life, how do you handle them?

Most of the time, is this way successful?

Value-Belief Pattern

Generally get things you want out of life?

Important things in your life?

If appropriate: Have important plans for the future?

Is religion important in your life?

If appropriate: Does this help when difficulties arise?

If appropriate: Will being here interfere with any religious practices?

(See Tab 13, Jarel Spiritual Well-Being Scale, for in-depth assessment.)
If patient is hospitalized: Things that are important to you while you are here?

Examination

Directions: Circle if present or describe the finding.

Health Perception–Health Management Pattern

Observe general appearance: Dressed appropriately to situation or disheveled: _____ Awake or drowsy: _____ Agitated or nervous: _____
Appearance consistent with health status described in history? _____

Nutritional-Metabolic Pattern

Body temperature _____ Skin: bony prominences? _____
Lesions? _____ Color changes? _____
Moistness? _____ Bruises? _____
If redness over bony prominence or pressure ulcer, see Braden Scale, Tab 4.
Take picture of any lesions over bony prominences at baseline.
Dryness, discomfort from calluses on feet?

Ankle edema _____ or rings on fingers unusually tight?

Oral mucous membranes: Color: _____ Moistness: _____
Lesions: _____
Teeth and gums: General appearance? _____
Alignment of teeth: _____ Dentures: _____
Cavities: _____ Missing teeth: _____
Abdominal distention? _____
_____
Actual weight: _____ Height _____
Body mass index: _____ Waist-to-hip ratio _____
Intravenous or other type of feeding? (Specify type.)
_____
_____

Elimination Pattern

If indicated: Examine excreta or drainage as to its color, amount, and
consistency:
_____
_____

Activity-Exercise Pattern

(Some assessment items are adapted from Morris [1990].)

Pulse (rate) _____ (rhythm) _____ (strength) _____
Blood pressure _____ Respiration rate _____
Rhythm _____ Depth _____
Breath sounds _____
Oxygen saturation (oximeter reading) _____
Hand grip strength: Normal _____ Weak _____ Strong _____
Muscle firmness (tone) _____
Range of motion: Joints _____
Motor function (check one):
   0: No impairment __
   1: Localized (specify location) __
   2: Impairment one side __
   3: Impairment both sides __
Absent body part (identify) __
Mobility (check one):
   Bedrest __
   Unable to move independently __
   Bed mobility: __
   While in bed, can turn side to side and position body __
   Ambulatory __
   Ambulatory with cane/walker/crutches __
   Wheelchair __
   Gait __

Posture _____
Balance _____
Demonstrated ability for (rate on functional levels scale; see Tab 6):
Feeding ____ Bathing _____ Dressing _____ Grooming _____ Toileting _____

Sleep-Rest Pattern
If appropriate (e.g., in hospital): Observe sleep pattern and, when awake,
physical appearance:
_____
_____

Cognitive-Perceptual Pattern
Orientation to time, place, and person:
_____
_____

Level of consciousness (If in coma, see Tab 8 for in-depth assessment):
_____
_____

Hears whisper? (Check right/left) Yes _____ No _____
Reads newsprint? Yes _____ No _____
Can pick up a pencil? Yes _____ No _____
Grasps ideas and questions during assessment (abstract, concrete)
Yes _____ No _____
Language spoken:
_____
Vocabulary level:
_____
Attention span (average to easily distracted):
_____
_____
Understanding of verbal messages (always, sometimes, rarely):
_____
_____

(If problem present, see Tab 8 for in-depth assessment.)
Decision Making

Self-Perception–Self-Concept Pattern
Eye contact: Yes _____ No _____
Confident manner (speech and appearance)? Use more than one encounter.
Yes _____ No _____
Posture/Dress/Grooming:
_____
_____
Attention span on a scale of 1 to 10, with 1 being attentive and 10 being
distracted: _____
Tension level on a scale of 1 to 10, with 1 being relaxed and 10 being
nervous: _____

Interpersonal manner on a scale of 1 to 10 with 1 being assertive and 10 being passive:

Interaction with family member or other (if present). Describe:

Role-Relationship Pattern
Interaction among family member(s) or others (if present). Describe (e.g., caring, supportive, blaming, argumentative, etc., or minimal opportunity for interaction):

Sexuality-Reproductive Pattern
None unless doing full physical examination.

Coping–Stress Tolerance Pattern
On a scale of 1 to 10, with 1 being relaxed and 10 being nervous, describe the patient:

Repeat after a time lapse.

Value-Belief Pattern
Note signs of worship (rosary, pictures, shawl, etc):

Family Assessment Guidelines*

Interview may be with entire family or just one member, usually a parent. If one member has a health problem and an assessment is indicated, use the Individual Assessment Guidelines.

History

Health Perception–Health Management Pattern
How has the family's general health been (in last few years)?

_____

*See individual or family guidelines to clarify information.

Family members had colds in the past year?

_____

Absences from work/school?

_____

Most important things family does to keep healthy?

_____

Think these make a difference to health? (Include family folk remedies, if appropriate.)

_____

Immunizations? (Include status of adults and children.)

_____

Have a regular health-care provider?

_____

Frequency of checkups?

_____

Adults?

_____

Children?

_____

If children in house: Storage of drugs and cleaning products?

_____

Disposal of drugs?

_____

Accidents in last few years (home, work, school, driving)?

_____

Use of scatter rugs in any room?

_____

In the past, has it been easy to find ways to carry out doctors' or nurses' suggestions?

_____

Other things in family's health that are of concern?

_____
_____

Nutritional-Metabolic Pattern

Typical family meal pattern/food intake, including supplements (e.g., vitamins, types of snacks):

_____

Typical family fluid intake, including types (e.g., fruit juices, soft drinks, coffee):

_____

Appetite?

_____

Problems?

_____

Dental care?

_____

Frequency?

_____

Skin or skin-healing problems?

_____

Elimination Pattern

Problems in waste/garbage disposal?

_____

Pet animals' waste disposal (indoor/outdoor)?

_____

If indicated: Problems with flies, roaches, rodents?

_____

Activity-Exercise Pattern

Any problems in: Shopping, including transportation to and from the store?

_____

Schedule-keeping for members (e.g., children's activities)?

_____

Cooking and meal preparation?

_____

Keeping up the house (e.g., cleaning, repairing)?

_____

Budgeting work/income for food, clothes, home, and other costs?

_____

Approximately how many hours per week do family members exercise?

_____

Type?

_____

Regularity?

_____

Family leisure activities? Active (e.g., sports, walking) or passive (e.g., television, computer games)?

_____

If relevant: Any difficulty managing care of dependent children, other?

_____

Sleep-Rest Pattern
Most days, do family members seem to be well rested and ready for school/work?

_____

Sufficient space and quiet, dark, sleeping area available?

_____

If relevant: Young baby in family? _____
Toddler asking to sleep in parent's bed?

_____

Family finds time to relax before sleep?

_____

Cognitive-Perceptual Pattern
Any member with visual or hearing problems? If so, how managed?

_____

Any important decisions family has had to make?

_____

How does family make important decisions?

Self-Perception–Self-Concept Pattern

Most of time family feels good about themselves as a family (support each other, feeling of love and closeness, sharing)?

General mood of family? Happy? Anxious? Depressed?

What helps family mood when "down"?

Role-Relationship Pattern
Family members living at home? Any extended family in close touch? Diagram relationships if relevant (see Genogram in Tab 10.)

Ages of members and family structure:

Any current family problem that is difficult to handle (nuclear/extended)?

If children/teenagers in family: Problems in child rearing?

Members respect privacy needs of family members?

Number of meals per day that family is able to eat together?

Participate in joint recreational activities?

Relationships good among family members? Among siblings? Between parents? Extended family?

Members support each other?

If appropriate: Income sufficient for needs?

Feel part of (or isolated from) community?

From neighbors?

Any adult, dependent members requiring care?

Who is the caregiver?

Problems providing care?

Sexuality-Reproductive Pattern

If appropriate (sexual partner within household or situation):
Are sexual relations satisfying? Any problems?

Elderly married: Any change in your and your wife's/husband's interest in sex?

Unmarried: Any problems regarding sex?

If appropriate: Use of family planning? Any problems?

If appropriate: Is it easy to find time and privacy for intimacy?

If appropriate (to age of children): Feel comfortable in explaining/discussing sexual subjects with your children?

If appropriate: Any children sexually active? Know about safe sex?

_____

Coping–Stress Tolerance Pattern
Any big changes (difficult situations) within family in last few years? If so, how members have adapted to change?

_____

Family tense or relaxed most of time?

_____

If tense, what helps?

_____

Anyone use medicines, drugs, or alcohol to decrease tension?

_____

When everyday family problems arise, how handled?

_____

Most of the time, is this way successful in resolving the problem?

_____

Family plan for communicating among members and managing an emergency?

_____

Value-Belief Pattern
Generally, family members get things they want out of life?

_____

Important things family is thinking about for the future?

_____

Any rules about behavior that family thinks are important?

_____

Religion important in family?

_____

If yes, does this help when difficulties arise?

_____

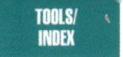

Examination

Health Perception–Health Management Pattern
General appearance of family members:

_____

If appropriate: Check medicine storage, cribs, playpens, stove, scatter rugs:

_____

Check home/yard safety hazards with family:

_____

(For in-depth assessment of home safety, see Tab 3, Home Environment Safety Checklist.)

Nutritional-Metabolic Pattern
If opportunity available: Check food types in pantry and refrigerator contents/temperature, meal preparation, contents of meal, etc.:

_____

Elimination Pattern
If opportunity available: Examine toilet facilities, garbage disposal, pet waste disposal, and indicators of risk for flies, roaches, and rodents:

_____

Activity-Exercise Pattern
General appearance: Home maintenance:

_____

Personal maintenance: Dressing, grooming of members present:

_____

Sleep-Rest Pattern
If opportunity available: Observe sleeping space and arrangements:

_____

Family members appear alert and well rested?

_____

Cognitive-Perceptual Pattern
If indicated: Language spoken at home:

Vocabulary level:

Grasp of ideas and questions (abstract/concrete):

Self-Perception–Self-Concept Pattern
General mood state: Relaxed (1) to nervous (5):

Members' response style: Passive (1) to assertive (5):

Role-Relationship Pattern
Interaction among family members (if present):

If opportunity: Observe family leadership roles. Which member(s) assume a leadership role? Observe leadership styles:

Sexuality-Reproductive Pattern
This pattern goes unexamined.

Coping–Stress Tolerance Pattern
This pattern goes unexamined unless there is an opportunity to observe stressor and stress management.

Value-Belief Pattern
Note signs of worship (crosses, rosary, pictures, shawl, etc.):

Community Assessment Guidelines*

Community representatives, including residents, families surveyed in the supermarket, staff of community health-care agencies, and public health department personnel, provide assessment information. Public documents, such as statistical health data, laws, and health department rules and regulations, also provide information.

*See individual or family assessment guidelines to clarify information.

History

Health Perception–Health Management Pattern
In general, what is the health/wellness level of the community on a scale of 1 to 5, with 5 being the highest?

Any major health problems?

Particular groups?

Any strong cultural patterns influencing health practices of groups in the area (e.g., immigrants, aged with traditional culture)?

Do people feel they have access to health services?

Demand for any particular health services or prevention programs?

Do people feel fire, police, safety programs sufficient?

Concerns with air pollution or soil, water, food contamination?

Nutritional-Metabolic Pattern
In general, do most people seem well nourished?

Children?

Adults?

Elderly?

Food supplement programs for low income?

School nutrition programs?

Foods reasonably priced in this geographic area relative to income?

Grocery and drug stores accessible to most people?

"Meals on Wheels" available?

Dental problems common?

Dental care accessible?

Water supply and quality?

Testing services (if most people have own wells)?

Restaurant food inspection programs?

If appropriate: Water usage cost?

Any drought restrictions?

Any concern that community growth will exceed good water supply?

Utility costs manageable for most households?

Programs to help low income?

TOOLS/
INDEX

Elimination Pattern

Major kinds of wastes (e.g., industrial, sewage)?
_____

Disposal systems?
_____

Recycling programs?
_____

Any problems perceived by community?
_____

Pest control?
_____

Food service inspection (e.g., restaurants, street vendors)?
_____

Activity-Exercise Pattern

Is transportation convenient and affordable for:
Work?
_____

Shopping?
_____

Recreation?
_____

Health care?
_____

People use community centers/playgrounds?
_____

Seniors?
_____

Children?
_____

Adults?
_____

Is housing adequate (availability, cost)?
_____

Low-income housing?
_____
_____

Senior housing?
_____
_____

Sleep-Rest Pattern
Generally quiet at night in most neighborhoods?
_____

Usual business hours?
_____

"Around-the-clock" industries?
_____
_____

Cognitive-Perceptual Pattern
Most groups speak English?
_____

Other predominant languages?
_____

Bilingual?
_____

Average educational level of people in the community?
_____
_____

Schools seen as good or need improving?
_____

Adult education desired?
_____

Available?
_____

Types of problems that require community decisions?
_____

Decision-making process?
_____
_____
_____

What is the best way to get things done/changed in this community?

Self-Perception–Self-Concept Pattern

Good community to live in?

Why?

Status going up, down, or staying about the same?

Old community? Fairly new?

Does any age group predominate?

People's mood in general: Enjoying life? Stressed? Depressed?

People generally have the kind of abilities needed in this community?

Community/neighborhood functions?

Parades/celebrations?

Picnics?

Role-Relationship Pattern

People seem to get along well together here?

Places where people go to socialize?

Do people feel government listens to them?

High/low participation at community meetings?

Enough work/jobs for everybody?

Wages good/fair?

Do people seem to like the kind of work available (happy in their jobs)?

Any problems with violence in the neighborhoods?

Family violence?

Problems with child/spouse/elder abuse?

Get along with adjacent communities?

Collaborate on any community projects?

Do neighbors seem to support each other?

Community get-togethers?

Sexuality-Reproductive Pattern
People feel there are problems with pornography, prostitution, adult book/-video stores?

Sufficient police protection and community education to prevent sexual violence?

Do people want/support sex education in schools/community?

Average family size?

Maternal and infant mortality rates?

Sufficient prenatal clinic facilities?

Coping–Stress Tolerance Pattern
Any recent community stress?

How handled?

Any current groups under stress or exhibiting tension?

Availability of phone help lines such as 911 and suicide help line?

Groups (health-related, other) trained to handle emergencies?

Value-Belief Pattern
Community values: Top four things that people living here see as important in their lives? Note the health-related values, priorities:

People tend to get involved in causes/local fund-raising campaigns? Note if any are health-related.

Religious groups in the community?

Places to worship available for all denominations?

People tolerant of cultural or religious differences?

Examination

Conduct your examination through observation of the community and an examination of public records.

Health Perception–Health Management Pattern
Morbidity, mortality, longevity, disability rates (by age groups and sex, if available):

_____

Accident rates (by district, if available):

_____

Hazardous conditions:

_____

Health facilities (types):

_____

Nursing home safety records (nurse/resident ratios, falls):

_____

Hospital infection rates:

_____

Ongoing health promotion/prevention programs (utilization rates):

_____

Ratio of health professionals to population:

_____

Percentage of people with health insurance:

_____

Laws regarding drinking age:

_____

Arrest statistics for drugs, drunk driving by age group:

_____

Incidence of HIV, AIDS, tuberculosis:

_____

Nutritional-Metabolic Pattern
General appearance of people (nutrition, teeth, clothing appropriate to climate):

Children:

Adults:

Elderly:

Food purchases (observations of food store check-out counters):

Availability of "junk" food machines (in schools, etc.):

Monitoring of water supply. Check quality:

Restaurant inspections:

Elimination Pattern
Communicable-disease statistics (water-borne, etc.):

Air pollution statistics:

Activity-Exercise Pattern
Recreation/cultural programs:

Availability of nursing homes:

Assistive living facilities:

Senior center with exercise, recreational programs:

Affordable housing:

Structural aids for the disabled (curbs, bathrooms):

Child care resources available:

Rehabilitation facilities:

External maintenance of streets, homes, yards, apartment houses:

Transportation services relative to need:

Sleep-Rest Pattern
Activity-noise levels in business district:

In residential district:

Noise regulations or laws:

Cognitive-Perceptual Pattern
Quality, number, location of school facilities:

School drop-out rate:

Adult education programs:

Community government structure; decision-making lines (organizational chart showing how decisions are made that affect health health-care services):

Percentage residents English-speaking:

Percentage residents speak English as second language:

English classes available?

Self-Perception–Self-Concept Pattern
Racial, ethnic mix:

Socioeconomic levels:

General observations of mood, within the community at large and in meetings:

Available mental health services relative to need:

Role-Relationship Pattern
Observation of interactions (among people in the supermarket or at specific meetings):

Statistics on personal or interpersonal crimes:

Statistics on employment:

Statistics on income/poverty:

Divorce rate:

Sexuality–Reproductive Pattern
Average family size and types of households (e.g., related or unrelated, single parent, both parents, single alone):

Male/female ratio:

Average maternal age:

Maternal mortality rate:

Infant mortality rate:

Teen pregnancy rate:

Divorce rate:

Abortion rate:

Sexual violence statistics:

Laws/regulations regarding information on birth control:

Statistics on sexually transmitted diseases:

Coping–Stress Tolerance Pattern
Statistics on social problems as measures of social stress:
Delinquency:

Drug abuse:

Alcoholism:

Suicide:

Psychiatric illness:

Suicide by age groups:

Teenage after-school recreation areas:

Unemployment rates by race/ethnic group/sex:

Emergency and disaster plans:

Designation of shelters and medical supplies (if needed for weather-related or other crisis):

Value-Belief Pattern
Zoning/conservation laws:

Scan of community government health committee reports (goals, priorities):

Health budget relative to total budget:

Parks, museums, concert programs for the public:

Places of worship (note if number relative to need):

Functional Health Pattern Screening Assessment (FHPSA)

- The FHPSA is based on Gordon's (1994) 11 Functional Health Patterns.
- The FHPSA includes 58 screening questions and represents all 11 functional health patterns.
- Additional questions can be added to the FHPSA to reflect a particular patient group.
- The patient can self-complete the FHPSA by circling the responses on a 4-point scale, with responses ranging from *never* or *does not occur* (1) to *routinely* or *occurs the majority of the time* (4).
- Nurses can quickly review patient responses and generate additional branching questions to more fully illuminate responses when needed.

- A research tool, the **Functional Health Pattern Assessment Screening Tool** (FHPAST), has also been developed (Jones, 2002). The psychometric properties have been developed to yield a 47-item research instrument with a three-factor solution. For more information, contact the authors directly at djones@partners.org or ffoster@partners.org

Directions Demographics

Below are a series of items designed to screen behaviors that affect your health. Please read each item, and circle one number for the response that best applies to you over the past **4** weeks.

Definition of Responses Demographics

1. Never *or* does not occur.
2. Sometimes *or* occurs sporadically.
3. Often *or* occurs occasionally but not on a routine basis.
4. Routinely *or* occurs the majority of the time.
   1. Age: _____
   2. Sex: F _____ M _____
   3. Race: _____
   4. Religion _____

Health Perception–Health Management Pattern				
I can make changes in lifestyle to improve my health.	1	2	3	4
I seek immediate attention for changes in my health.	1	2	3	4
I have an annual health examination.	1	2	3	4
I am able to follow recommendations from my health-care provider.	1	2	3	4
I wear a seat belt.	1	2	3	4
I am in excellent health.	1	2	3	4
I consider myself to be healthy.	1	2	3	4
When I drink alcohol, wine, or beer, I feel guilty.	1	2	3	4
I use recreational drugs.	1	2	3	4
I smoke cigarettes.	1	2	3	4
I feel at risk for physical harm.	1	2	3	4
Nutritional-Metabolic Pattern				
I intentionally limit my dietary intake of fat.	1	2	3	4
I feel comfortable with my weight.	1	2	3	4

I heal easily.	1	2	3	4
I avoid the sun or use sunscreen.	1	2	3	4
I eat 5–6 servings of fruits and vegetables each day.	1	2	3	4
I drink 6–8 glasses of water a day.	1	2	3	4
Elimination Pattern				
I have difficulty urinating.	1	2	3	4
I have problems with bowel elimination.	1	2	3	4
Activity-Exercise Pattern				
I have enough energy for my daily activities.	1	2	3	4
I do aerobic exercise for at least 20 minutes three or more times a week.	1	2	3	4
My physical abilities limit my daily activities.	1	2	3	4
I feel unusual physical symptoms with walking.	1	2	3	4
Sleep-Rest Pattern				
I feel rested when I awake.	1	2	3	4
I fall to sleep without a problem.	1	2	3	4
Cognitive-Perceptual Pattern				
I feel good about the decisions I make.	1	2	3	4
I am satisfied with my ability to solve problems.	1	2	3	4
I am able to hear clearly.	1	2	3	4
I am able to concentrate for a long period of time.	1	2	3	4
I am able to learn new information easily.	1	2	3	4
The choices I make about my life are consistent with my values.	1	2	3	4
I have difficulty with my vision.	1	2	3	4
I experience pain that interrupts my daily activities.	1	2	3	4
Self-Perception–Self-Concept Pattern				
I feel good about myself.	1	2	3	4
I feel comfortable with my weight.	1	2	3	4
I feel hopeful about the future.	1	2	3	4

I feel like I am in control of my life.	1	2	3	4
I like the way I look.	1	2	3	4
I am happy with my life.	1	2	3	4
I worry a lot.	1	2	3	4
I fear for my safety.	1	2	3	4
Role-Relationship Pattern				
I am satisfied with what I do for work.	1	2	3	4
I feel comfortable with the role I play in my family.	1	2	3	4
I am satisfied with my social life.	1	2	3	4
I feel comfortable expressing my feelings and emotions.	1	2	3	4
I feel I can easily communicate with others.	1	2	3	4
It is a burden to participate in family caretaking activities.	1	2	3	4
I feel at risk for physical harm.	1	2	3	4
I have family problems that I find are difficult to handle.	1	2	3	4
Sexuality-Reproductive Pattern				
When I am sexually active, I am at low risk for getting a sexually transmitted disease.	1	2	3	4
I am comfortable with my sexuality.	1	2	3	4
Coping–Stress Tolerance Pattern				
I am able to cope with the stresses in my life.	1	2	3	4
I have someone I can talk to when I need help or support.	1	2	3	4
I am able to adjust to changes in my life.	1	2	3	4
I have a usual routine that I perform to help me relax.	1	2	3	4
I experience physical discomfort when I am under stress.	1	2	3	4
I feel stress, tension, or pressure.	1	2	3	4

Value-Belief Pattern				
Religious or spiritual practices give meaning to my life.	1	2	3	4
My health is important to me.				
The choices I make about my life are consistent with my values.	1	2	3	4

Foster & Jones, 1997–2004, with permission.

Diagnostic Categories Grouped by Functional Health Patterns, 2006–2008

Plain type indicates diagnoses currently accepted by NANDA International. Blue type indicates diagnoses developed by the author or others, not yet reviewed by NANDA, but are found to be useful in clinical practice.

Health Perception–Health Management Pattern

- Health-Seeking Behaviors (Specify)
- Risk-Prone Health Behavior
- Ineffective Health Maintenance (Specify Area)
- Ineffective Therapeutic Regimen Management (Specify Area)
- Risk for Ineffective Therapeutic Regimen Management (Specify Area)
- Effective Therapeutic Regimen Management
- Readiness for Enhanced Therapeutic Regimen Management
- Ineffective Family Therapeutic Regimen Management
- Ineffective Community Therapeutic Regimen Management
- Noncompliance (Specify Area)
- Risk for Noncompliance (Specify Area)
- Contamination
- Risk for Contamination
- Readiness for Enhanced Immunization Status
- Risk for Infection (Specify Type/Area)
- Risk for Injury (Trauma)
- Risk for Falls
- Risk for Perioperative-Positioning Injury
- Risk for Poisoning
- Risk for Suffocation
- Ineffective Protection (Specify)
- Disturbed Energy Field

Nutritional-Metabolic Pattern

- Failure to Thrive (Adult)
- Imbalanced Nutrition: More than Body Requirements or Exogenous Obesity
- Imbalanced Nutrition: Risk for More than Body Requirements or Risk for Obesity
- Imbalanced Nutrition: Less than Body Requirements or Nutritional Deficit (Specify Type)
- Readiness for Enhanced Nutrition
- Interrupted Breastfeeding
- Ineffective Breastfeeding
- Effective Breastfeeding
- Ineffective Infant Feeding Pattern
- Impaired Swallowing (Uncompensated)
- Nausea
- Risk for Aspiration
- Impaired Oral Mucous Membrane
- Impaired Dentition
- Risk for Imbalanced Fluid Volume
- Excess Fluid Volume
- Deficient Fluid Volume
- Risk for Deficient Fluid Volume
- Readiness for Enhanced Fluid Volume
- Impaired Skin Integrity
- Risk for Impaired Skin Integrity
- Impaired Tissue Integrity (Specify Type)
- Pressure Ulcer (Specify Stage)
- Latex Allergy Response
- Risk for Latex Allergy Response
- Ineffective Thermoregulation
- Hyperthermia
- Hypothermia
- Risk for Imbalanced Body Temperature
- Risk for Impaired Liver Function
- Risk for Unstable Blood Glucose

Elimination Pattern

- Constipation
- Perceived Constipation
- Intermittent Constipation

- Risk for Constipation
- Diarrhea
- Bowel Incontinence
- Impaired Urinary Elimination
- Readiness for Enhanced Urinary Elimination
- Functional Urinary Incontinence
- Overflow Urinary Incontinence
- Reflex Urinary Incontinence
- Stress Urinary Incontinence
- Urge Urinary Incontinence
- Risk for Urge Urinary Incontinence
- Total Urinary Incontinence
- Urinary Retention

Activity-Exercise Pattern

- Activity Intolerance (Specify Level)
- Risk for Activity Intolerance
- Fatigue
- Sedentary Lifestyle
- Deficient Diversional Activity
- Impaired Physical Mobility (Specify Level)
- Impaired Wheelchair Mobility
- Impaired Bed Mobility (Specify Level)
- Impaired Transfer Ability (Specify Level)
- Impaired Walking (Specify Level)
- Wandering
- Risk for Disuse Syndrome
- Risk for Joint Contractures
- Total Self-Care Deficit (Specify Level)
- Bathing-Hygiene Self-Care Deficit (Specify Level)
- Dressing-Grooming Self-Care Deficit (Specify Level)
- Feeding Self-Care Deficit (Specify Level)
- Toileting Self-Care Deficit (Specify Level)
- Developmental Delay: Self-Care Skills (Specify Level)
- Readiness for Enhanced Self-Care
- Delayed Surgical Recovery
- Delayed Growth and Development
- Risk for Delayed Development
- Risk for Disproportionate Growth
- Impaired Home Maintenance
- Dysfunctional Ventilatory Weaning Response (DVWR)
- Impaired Spontaneous Ventilation

- Ineffective Airway Clearance
- Ineffective Breathing Pattern
- Impaired Gas Exchange
- Decreased Cardiac Output
- Ineffective Tissue Perfusion (Specify Type)
- Autonomic Dysreflexia
- Risk for Autonomic Dysreflexia
- Risk for Sudden Infant Death Syndrome
- Disorganized Infant Behavior
- Risk for Disorganized Infant Behavior
- Readiness for Enhanced Organized Infant Behavior
- Risk for Peripheral Neurovascular Dysfunction
- Decreased Intracranial Adaptive Capacity

Sleep-Rest Pattern

- Insomnia
- Delayed Sleep Onset
- Sleep Deprivation
- Sleep Pattern Reversal
- Readiness for Enhanced Sleep

Cognitive-Perceptual Pattern

- Acute Pain (Specify Type and Location)
- Chronic Pain (Specify Type and Location)
- Pain Self-Management Deficit (Acute, Chronic)
- Readiness for Enhanced Comfort
- Disturbed Sensory Perception (Specify)
- Uncompensated Sensory Loss (Specify Type/Degree)
- Sensory Overload Effects
- Sensory Deprivation Effects
- Unilateral Neglect
- Deficient Knowledge (Specify Area)
- Readiness for Enhanced Knowledge
- Disturbed Thought Processes (Specify)
- Attention-Concentration Deficit
- Acute Confusion
- Risk for Acute Confusion
- Chronic Confusion
- Impaired Environmental Interpretation Syndrome
- Impaired Memory

- Risk for Cognitive Impairment
- Readiness for Enhanced Decision-Making
- Decisional Conflict (Specify)

Self-Perception–Self-Concept Pattern

- Fear (Specify Focus)
- Anxiety
- Mild Anxiety
- Moderate Anxiety
- Severe Anxiety (Panic)
- Anticipatory Anxiety (Mild, Moderate, Severe)
- Death Anxiety
- Reactive Depression (Specify Situation)
- Risk for Loneliness
- Hopelessness
- Risk for Self-Directed Violence
- Readiness for Enhanced Hope
- Powerlessness (Severe, Moderate, Low)
- Risk for Powerlessness
- Readiness for Enhanced Power
- Risk for Compromised Human Dignity
- Chronic Low Self-Esteem
- Situational Low Self-Esteem
- Risk for Situational Low Self-Esteem
- Readiness for Enhanced Self-Concept
- Disturbed Body Image
- Disturbed Personal Identity

Role-Relationship Pattern

- Grieving
- Anticipatory Grieving
- Complicated Grieving
- Risk for Complicated Grieving
- Chronic Sorrow
- Ineffective Role Performance
- Unresolved Independence-Dependence Conflict
- Social Isolation or Social Rejection
- Social Isolation
- Impaired Social Interaction
- Developmental Delay: Social Skills (Specify)

- Relocation Stress Syndrome
- Risk for Relocation Stress Syndrome
- Interrupted Family Processes (Specify)
- Dysfunctional Family Process: Alcoholism
- Impaired Parenting (Specify Alteration)
- Risk for Impaired Parenting (Specify Alteration)
- Parental Role Conflict
- Weak Parent-Infant Attachment
- Risk for Impaired Parent-Infant/Child Attachment
- Parent-Infant Separation*
- Readiness for Enhanced Parenting
- Readiness for Enhanced Family Processes
- Caregiver Role Strain
- Risk for Caregiver Role Strain
- Impaired Verbal Communication
- Developmental Delay: Communication Skills
- Readiness for Enhanced Communication
- Risk for Other-Directed Violence

Sexuality-Reproductive Pattern

- Ineffective Sexuality Patterns
- Sexual Dysfunction
- Rape Trauma Syndrome
- Rape Trauma Syndrome: Compound Reaction
- Rape Trauma Syndrome: Silent Reaction

Coping—Stress Tolerance Pattern

- Ineffective Coping
- Avoidance Coping
- Defensive Coping
- Ineffective Denial or Denial
- Readiness for Enhanced Coping
- Risk for Suicide
- Stress Overload
- Readiness for Enhanced Family Coping
- Compromised Family Coping
- Disabled Family Coping
- Ineffective Community Coping
- Readiness for Enhanced Community Coping

*The diagnosis Parent-Infant Separation was developed by T. Heather Herdman, Ph.D., R.N. Clinical Nurse Specialist, based on her research in neonatal intensive care.

- Support System Deficit
- Post-Trauma Syndrome
- Risk for Post-Trauma Syndrome
- Self-Mutilation
- Risk for Self-Mutilation

Value-Belief Pattern

- Moral Distress
- Spiritual Distress (Distress of Human Spirit)
- Risk for Spiritual Distress
- Readiness for Enhanced Spiritual Well-Being
- Impaired Religiosity
- Risk for Impaired Religiosity
- Readiness for Enhanced Religiosity

Screening Assessment

When it is not possible to do an assessment on admission, a screening assessment may be indicated. The following are some suggested items.

History

Health Perception–Health Management Pattern
Any general health concerns?
_____
_____

Taking any medications? (List name, dosage, time taken.)
_____

Bring these with you?
_____

Allergies? List.
_____
_____

Nutritional-Metabolic Pattern
Any dietary restrictions?
_____
_____

Problems swallowing, digesting?

Elimination Pattern
Problems in moving bowels, passing urine?

Activity-Exercise Pattern
Any activity restrictions? Problems walking?

Shortness of breath?

Leg cramps?

Sleep-Rest Pattern
Most mornings feel rested and ready to go?

Cognitive-Perceptual Pattern
Pain?

Orientation to place, person?

Vision problems? Wear glasses?

Hearing problems?

Self-Perception–Self-Concept Pattern
Feeling nervous or anxious?

Role-Relationship Pattern
Anyone depending on you at home?

Sexuality-Reproductive Pattern
Deferred unless relevant to medical condition.

Coping–Stress Tolerance Pattern
Someone you would want to call?

Value-Belief Pattern
Any other things important to you?

Wish to have someone from your religion visit?

Examination

Inspect skin:

Check safety of ambulation:

Evaluate mood state (anxious, depressed):

Nursing Specialty Assessment

Awareness of frequently occurring problems increases the nurse's sensitivity to cues during assessment. The following are examples of nursing diagnoses in specialty practice that will guide in-depth assessment when using assessment guidelines.

Geriatric Nursing

Diagnoses reflect the literature in this specialty.

Health Perception–Health Management Pattern
- Health-Seeking Behaviors
- Risk for Ineffective Health Management
- Ineffective Management of Therapeutic Regimen
- Noncompliance (Specify Area)
- Risk for Noncompliance
- Risk for Injury
- Risk for Falls
- Risk for Infection

Nutritional-Metabolic Pattern
- Nutritional Deficit
- Impaired Dentition
- Deficient Fluid Volume
- Impaired Swallowing
- Risk for Impaired Skin Integrity

Elimination Pattern
- Incontinence (see types)
- Constipation

Activity-Exercise Pattern
- Risk for Activity Intolerance
- Activity Intolerance
- Impaired Mobility
- Self-Care Deficits
- Deficient Diversional Activity
- Impaired Home Maintenance
- Fatigue
- Impaired Walking

Sleep-Rest Pattern
- Sleep Pattern Reversal
- Insomnia
- Delayed Sleep Onset

Cognitive-Perceptual Pattern
- Chronic Pain
- Joint Pain
- Confusion
- Impaired Memory
- Sensory Loss (Vision, Hearing, Touch, Smell)

Self-Perception–Self-Concept Pattern
- Fear (Specify)
- Anxiety
- Reactive Situational Depression (Specify)
- Risk for Loneliness
- Powerlessness
- Disturbed Body Image
- Low Self-Esteem

Role-Relationship Pattern
- Chronic Sorrow
- Risk for Caregiver Role Strain
- Caregiver Role Strain
- Relocation Syndrome

Sexuality-Reproductive Pattern
- Sexual Dysfunction

Coping–Stress Tolerance Pattern
- Support System Deficit
- Ineffective Coping

Value-Belief Pattern
- Spiritual Distress
- Readiness for Enhanced Spiritual Well-Being
- Risk for Spiritual Distress

Rehabilitation Nursing

Over 700 members of the American Rehabilitation Nurses Association rated 145 nursing diagnoses. Diagnoses rated as nearly always or frequently present in their practice are the following (from Gordon, 1995):

Health Perception–Health Management Pattern
- Risk for Injury or Falls

Nutritional-Metabolic Pattern
- Risk for Impaired Skin Integrity
- Impaired Swallowing

Activity-Exercise Pattern
- Impaired Mobility
- Impaired Transfer Ability
- Impaired Locomotion (wheelchair)
- Impaired Walking

- Activity Intolerance
- Self-Care Deficit

Cognitive-Perceptual Pattern
- Deficient Knowledge
- Acute and Chronic Pain

Role-Relationship Pattern
- Impaired Verbal Communication

Rehabilitation Subspecialties

Additional diagnoses in the subspecialties are:

Stroke
- Unilateral Neglect
- Risk for Aspiration
- Impaired Bed Mobility
- Risk for Cognitive Impairment

Head Injury
- Disturbed Thought Processes
- Risk for Cognitive Impairment
- Attention-Concentration Deficit

Spinal Cord Injury
- Risk for Pressure Ulcer
- Bowel Incontinence
- Ineffective Sexuality Pattern
- Sexual Dysfunction
- Risk for Dysreflexia
- Risk for Infection

Critical Care Nursing

Unstable patients do not have the energy to tolerate a full history and examination until after discharge from the unit. There are common diagnoses, however, that should not be missed at the initial assessment. (Diagnoses are based in part on Gordon, 1992.)

Health Perception–Health Management Pattern
- Risk for Infection
- Risk for Injury
- Risk for Suffocation

Nutritional-Metabolic Pattern
- Risk for Nutritional Deficit
- Fluid Volume Deficit
- Risk for Pressure Ulcer
- Ineffective Thermoregulation

Elimination Pattern
- Risk for Constipation
- Total Incontinence

Activity-Exercise Pattern
- Risk for Activity Intolerance
- Self-Care Deficit (Levels 3 to 4)
- Risk for Joint Contractures
- Ineffective Airway Clearance

Sleep-Rest Pattern
- Delayed Sleep Onset
- Interrupted Sleep Pattern
- Sleep Deprivation

Cognitive-Perceptual Pattern
- Acute Pain
- Sensory Deprivation or Overload
- Risk for Cognitive Impairment
- Acute or Chronic Confusion
- Risk for Acute Confusion
- Decisional Conflict

Self-Perception–Self-Concept Pattern
- Fear (Specify)
- Anxiety
- Death Anxiety
- Powerlessness
- Self-Esteem Disturbance
- Disturbed Body Image

Role-Relationship Pattern
- Anticipatory Grieving
- Unresolved Independence-Dependence Conflict
- Altered Family Processes
- Impaired Communication

Coping–Stress Tolerance Pattern
- Ineffective Family Coping
- Avoidance Coping
- Denial

Value-Belief Pattern
- Spiritual Distress
- Risk for Spiritual Distress

Common Collaborative Problems: Critical Care

- Decreased Cardiac Output
- Impaired Gas Exchange
- Ineffective Tissue Perfusion
- Deficient or Excess Fluid Volume
- Imbalanced Fluid Volume
- Risk for Unstable Blood Glucose

Short-Stay Units

Most of the time it is not appropriate to obtain a full history in a recovery, labor and delivery, operating, or emergency room or in a walk-in clinic. In these cases, a screening assessment is used. If persons come to an emergency room with a nonemergent problem, nursing judgment will dictate the extent of assessment that is needed prior to referral or discharge to home. Diagnoses in short-stay units vary with the condition.

Diagnostic Categories* Grouped by Functional Health Patterns and Individual, Family, Community

Use this grouping of nursing diagnoses to describe assessment data when a functional pattern does not meet a standard or normative value. The following nursing diagnoses from the NANDA International Taxonomy II (2007) describe diagnostic judgments. Blue type indicates diagnoses developed by the author, not yet reviewed by NANDA, but found useful in clinical practice (Gordon, 2006).

Individual

Health Perception–Health Management Pattern
- Health-Seeking Behaviors (Specify)
- Risk-Prone Health Behavior
- Ineffective Health Management (Specify Area)

---

*From NANDA International (2005) NANDA Nursing Diagnoses: Definitions and Classification, 2005–2006, Philadelphia. Diagnoses in blue type from Gordon, M (2006) *Manual of Nursing Diagnosis,* 10th Edition, St Louis: Mosby.

- Ineffective Therapeutic Regimen Management (Specify Area)
- Risk for Ineffective Therapeutic Regimen Management (Specify Area)
- Effective Therapeutic Regimen Management
- Readiness for Enhanced Therapeutic Regimen Management
- Noncompliance (Specify Area)
- Risk for Noncompliance (Specify Area)
- Contamination
- Risk for Contamination
- Readiness for Enhanced Immunization Status
- Risk for Infection (Specify Type/Area)
- Risk for Injury (Trauma)
- Risk for Falls
- Risk for Perioperative-Positioning Injury
- Risk for Poisoning
- Risk for Suffocation
- Ineffective Protection (Specify)
- Disturbed Energy Field

Nutritional-Metabolic Pattern

- Failure to Thrive (Adult)
- Imbalanced Nutrition: More than Body Requirements or Exogenous Obesity
- Imbalanced Nutrition: Risk for More than Body Requirements or Risk for Obesity
- Imbalanced Nutrition: Less than Body Requirements or Nutritional Deficit (Specify Type)
- Readiness for Enhanced Nutrition
- Interrupted Breastfeeding
- Ineffective Breastfeeding
- Effective Breastfeeding
- Ineffective Infant Feeding Pattern
- Impaired Swallowing (Uncompensated)
- Nausea
- Risk for Aspiration
- Impaired Oral Mucous Membrane
- Impaired Dentition
- Imbalanced Fluid Volume
- Risk for Imbalanced Fluid Volume
- Excess Fluid Volume
- Deficient Fluid Volume
- Risk for Deficient Fluid Volume
- Readiness for Enhanced Fluid Volume
- Impaired Skin Integrity
- Risk for Impaired Skin Integrity

- ■ Impaired Tissue Integrity (Specify Type)
- ■ Pressure Ulcer (Specify Stage)
- ■ Latex Allergy Response
- ■ Risk for Latex Allergy Response
- ■ Ineffective Thermoregulation
- ■ Hyperthermia
- ■ Hypothermia
- ■ Risk for Imbalanced Body Temperature
- ■ Risk for Impaired Liver Function
- ■ Risk for Unstable Blood Glucose

Elimination Pattern
- ■ Constipation
- ■ Perceived Constipation
- ■ Intermittent Constipation
- ■ Risk for Constipation
- ■ Diarrhea
- ■ Bowel Incontinence
- ■ Impaired Urinary Elimination
- ■ Readiness for Enhanced Urinary Elimination
- ■ Functional Urinary Incontinence
- ■ Overflow Urinary incontinence
- ■ Reflex Urinary Incontinence
- ■ Stress Urinary Incontinence
- ■ Urge Urinary Incontinence
- ■ Risk for Urge Urinary Incontinence
- ■ Total Urinary Incontinence
- ■ Urinary Retention

Activity-Exercise Pattern
- ■ Activity Intolerance (Specify Level)
- ■ Risk for Activity Intolerance
- ■ Fatigue
- ■ Sedentary Lifestyle
- ■ Deficient Diversional Activity
- ■ Impaired Physical Mobility (Specify Level)
- ■ Impaired Wheelchair Mobility
- ■ Impaired Bed Mobility (Specify Level)
- ■ Impaired Transfer Ability (Specify Level)
- ■ Impaired Walking (Specify Level)
- ■ Wandering
- ■ Risk for Disuse Syndrome
- ■ Risk for Joint Contractures
- ■ Total Self-Care Deficit (Specify Level)

- Bathing-Hygiene Self-Care Deficit (Specify Level)
- Dressing-Grooming Self-Care Deficit (Specify Level)
- Feeding Self-Care Deficit (Specify Level)
- Toileting Self-Care Deficit (Specify Level)
- Developmental Delay: Self-Care Skills (Specify Level)
- Readiness for Enhanced Self-Care
- Delayed Surgical Recovery
- Delayed Growth and Development
- Risk for Delayed Development
- Risk for Disproportionate Growth
- Impaired Home Maintenance
- Dysfunctional Ventilatory Weaning Response (DVWR)
- Impaired Spontaneous Ventilation
- Ineffective Airway Clearance
- Ineffective Breathing Pattern
- Impaired Gas Exchange
- Decreased Cardiac Output
- Ineffective Tissue Perfusion (Specify Type)
- Autonomic Dysreflexia
- Risk for Autonomic Dysreflexia
- Risk for Sudden Infant Death Syndrome
- Disorganized Infant Behavior
- Risk for Disorganized Infant Behavior
- Readiness for Enhanced Organized Infant Behavior
- Risk for Peripheral Neurovascular Dysfunction
- Decreased Intracranial Adaptive Capacity

Sleep-Rest Pattern

- Insomnia
- Delayed Sleep Onset
- Sleep Deprivation
- Sleep Pattern Reversal
- Readiness for Enhanced Sleep

Cognitive-Perceptual Pattern

- Acute Pain (Specify Type and Location)
- Chronic Pain (Specify Type and Location)
- Pain Self-Management Deficit (Acute, Chronic)
- Readiness for Enhanced Comfort
- Disturbed Sensory Perception (Specify)
- Uncompensated Sensory Loss (Specify Type/Degree)
- Sensory Overload Effects
- Sensory Deprivation Effects
- Unilateral Neglect

- Deficient Knowledge (Specify Area)
- Readiness for Enhanced Knowledge
- Disturbed Thought Processes (Specify)
- Attention-Concentration Deficit
- Acute Confusion
- Risk for Acute Confusion
- Chronic Confusion
- Impaired Environmental Interpretation Syndrome
- Impaired Memory
- Risk for Cognitive Impairment
- Readiness for Enhanced Decision-Making
- Decisional Conflict (Specify)

Self-Perception–Self-Concept Pattern
- Fear (Specify Focus)
- Anxiety
- Mild Anxiety
- Moderate Anxiety
- Severe Anxiety (Panic)
- Anticipatory Anxiety (Mild, Moderate, Severe)
- Death Anxiety
- Reactive Depression (Specify Situation)
- Risk for Loneliness
- Hopelessness
- Risk for Self-Directed Violence
- Readiness for Enhanced Hope
- Powerlessness (Severe, Moderate, Low)
- Risk for Powerlessness
- Readiness for Enhanced Power
- Risk for Compromised Human Dignity
- Chronic Low Self-Esteem
- Situational Low Self-Esteem
- Risk for Situational Low Self-Esteem
- Readiness for Enhanced Self-Concept
- Disturbed Body Image
- Disturbed Personal Identity

Role-Relationship Pattern
- Grieving
- Anticipatory Grieving
- Complicated Grieving
- Risk for Complicated Grieving
- Chronic Sorrow
- Ineffective Role Performance

- Unresolved Independence-Dependence Conflict
- Social Isolation or Social Rejection
- Social Isolation
- Impaired Social Interaction
- Developmental Delay: Social Skills (Specify)
- Relocation Stress Syndrome
- Risk for Relocation Stress Syndrome
- Impaired Parenting (Specify Alteration)
- Risk for Impaired Parenting (Specify Alteration)
- Parental Role Conflict
- Weak Parent-Infant Attachment
- Risk for Impaired Parent-Infant/Child Attachment
- Parent-Infant Separation
- Readiness for Enhanced Parenting
- Caregiver Role Strain
- Risk for Caregiver Role Strain
- Impaired Verbal Communication
- Developmental Delay: Communication Skills
- Readiness for Enhanced Communication
- Risk for Other-Directed Violence

Sexuality-Reproductive Pattern
- Ineffective Sexuality Patterns
- Sexual Dysfunction
- Rape Trauma Syndrome
- Rape Trauma Syndrome: Compound Reaction
- Rape Trauma Syndrome: Silent Reaction

Coping–Stress Tolerance Pattern
- Ineffective Coping
- Avoidance Coping
- Defensive Coping
- Ineffective Denial or Denial
- Risk for Suicide
- Stress Overload
- Support System Deficit
- Post-Trauma Syndrome
- Risk for Post-Trauma Syndrome
- Self-Mutilation
- Risk for Self-Mutilation

Value-Belief Pattern
- Moral Distress
- Spiritual Distress (Distress of Human Spirit)
- Risk for Spiritual Distress

- Readiness for Enhanced Spiritual Well-Being
- Risk for Spiritual Distress
- Impaired Religiosity
- Risk for Impaired Religiosity
- Readiness for Enhanced Religiosity

Family Diagnoses

- Interrupted Family Processes (Specify)
- Dysfunctional Family Process: Alcoholism
- Readiness for Enhanced Family Processes
- Ineffective Family Therapeutic Regimen Management
- Readiness for Enhanced Family Coping
- Compromised Family Coping
- Disabled Family Coping

Community Diagnoses

- Ineffective Community Therapeutic Regimen Management
- Ineffective Community Coping
- Readiness for Enhanced Community Coping

Diagnoses Describing Risk States, 2006–2008

The following nursing diagnoses from the NANDA International Taxonomy II (2007) are used to describe diagnostic judgments. Blue type indicates diagnoses developed by the author, not yet reviewed by NANDA, but found useful in clinical practice (Gordon, 2006).

- Activity Intolerance, Risk for
- Allergy Response, Risk for Latex
- Aspiration, Risk for
- Attachment, Risk for Impaired Parent/Child
- Anxiety, Risk for Anticipatory
- Confusion, Risk for Acute
- Cognitive Impairment, Risk for
- Constipation, Risk for
- Contamination, Risk for
- Contractures, Risk for Joint
- Dignity, Risk for Compromised Human
- Disuse Syndrome, Risk for
- Dysreflexia, Risk for Autonomic
- Falls, Risk for

- Fluid Volume, Risk for Deficient
- Fluid Volume, Risk for Imbalanced
- Glucose, Risk for Unstable Blood
- Grieving, Risk for Complicated
- Growth, Risk for Disproportionate
- Incontinence, Risk for Urinary Urge
- Infant Behavior, Risk for Disorganized
- Infant Death Syndrome, Risk for Sudden
- Infection, Risk for
- Injury, Risk for
- Injury, Risk for Peri-operative-Positioning
- Liver Function, Risk for Impaired
- Loneliness, Risk for
- Noncompliance, Risk for
- Nutrition, Imbalanced: Risk for More Than Body Requirements
- Parenting, Risk for Impaired
- Peripheral Neurovascular Dysfunction, Risk for
- Poisoning, Risk for
- Post-Trauma Syndrome, Risk for
- Powerlessness, Risk for
- Religiosity, Risk for
- Relocation Stress Syndrome, Risk for
- Role Strain, Risk for Caregiver
- Self-Esteem, Risk for Situational Low
- Self-Mutilation, Risk for
- Skin Integrity, Risk for Impaired
- Spiritual Distress, Risk for
- Suffocation, Risk for
- Suicide, Risk for
- Temperature, Risk for Imbalanced Body
- Therapeutic Regimen Management, Risk for Ineffective
- Trauma, Risk for
- Violence, Risk for Other-Directed
- Violence, Risk for Self-Directed

Diagnoses Describing Wellness and Health, 2006–2008

The following nursing diagnoses from the NANDA International Taxonomy II (2007) describe diagnostic judgments.

- Communication, Readiness for Enhanced
- Coping, Readiness for Enhanced
- Fluid Balance, Readiness for Enhanced

- Infant Behavior, Readiness for Enhanced Organized
- Knowledge (Specify), Readiness for Enhanced
- Nutrition, Readiness for Enhanced
- Parenting, Readiness for Enhanced
- Self-Care, Readiness for Enhanced
- Self-Concept, Readiness for Enhanced
- Sleep, Readiness for Enhanced
- Spiritual Well-Being, Readiness for Enhanced
- Therapeutic Regimen Management, Readiness for Enhanced
- Urinary Elimination, Readiness for Enhanced
- Effective Breastfeeding
- Religiosity, Readiness for Enhanced

Diagnosis-Intervention-Outcome Links

The following are examples of diagnosis-intervention-outcome links for some common conditions. The content is from NANDA I (2007), Nursing Intervention Classification (Dochterman & Bulechek, 2004), the Nursing Outcome Classification, and NANDA, NOC, and NIC Linkages (Johnson, et al., 2006) with minimal changes.

- **75-year-old retired woman, former secretary living in inner-city neighborhood**

SOCIAL ISOLATION RELATED TO FEAR (STREET VIOLENCE)

- **Definition, Social Isolation:** Aloneness experienced by the individual and seen as a negative state.
- **Definition, Fear (Street Violence):** Perceived threat that is consciously recognized as a danger.

OUTCOME

- **Social Involvement:** Social interaction with persons, groups, or organizations.
- **Social Support:** Perceived availability and actual provision of reliable assistance from others.

INTERVENTIONS

- **Security Enhancement:** Intensifying a patient's sense of physical and psychological safety.
- **Anxiety and Fear Reduction:** Minimizing apprehension, dread, foreboding, or uneasiness related to anticipated danger.
- **Elder Support:** Facilitation of instrumental support and companionship in activities.

35-year-old actor with AIDS
RISK FOR SKIN INFECTION

■ **Definition:** Increased risk for being invaded by pathogenic organisms.

OUTCOME

■ **Infection Severity**

INTERVENTIONS

■ **Infection Control:** Minimizing the acquisition and transmission of infectious agents.
■ **Health-Promoting Behavior:** Personal actions to prevent infection.

50-year-old computer technician with knee surgery
IMPAIRED PHYSICAL MOBILITY RELATED TO ACUTE PAIN (POST-KNEE JOINT REPLACEMENT)

■ **Definition, Impaired Physical Mobility:** Limitation in independent, purposeful physical movement of the body or one or more extremities.
■ **Definition, Acute Pain:** Unpleasant sensory and emotional experience arising from actual or potential tissue damage or described in terms of such damage (International Association for the Study of Pain).

OUTCOME

■ Extent of positive perception of physical and psychological ease.

INTERVENTIONS

■ **Pain Management:** Alleviation or reduction in pain to a level of comfort that is acceptable to the patient.
■ **Positioning:** Deliberative placement of a body part to promote physiological and or psychological well-being.

References

American Nurses Association. (2000). *Standards of Clinical Nursing Practice.* Washington, DC: American Nurses Association.

Anderson J, et al. (2007). What you can learn from a comprehensive skin assessment. *Nursing 2007*, 37: 65–66.

Anno NJ. (1974). Behavioral treatment of sexual problems. Honolulu, Hawaii: Enabling Systems.

Barrett F & Jones D. (1999). Development and testing of functional health pattern assessment screening tool. In Rantz M & LeMone P (Eds.). *Proceedings of the 13th North American Diagnoses Association.* CINAHL Information Systems, Glendale, Calif.

Benson H, et al. (2006). Study of therapeutic effects of intercessory prayer (STEP) in cardiac bypass patients: A multi-center randomized trial of uncertainty and certainty of receiving intercessory prayer. *American Heart Journal,* 15(4): 934–942.

Borg GA. (1982). Borg scale. *Medicine and Science in Sports Exercise* 14: 377–387.

Chesson AL, et al. (1999). Practice parameters for the nonpharmacologic treatment of chronic insomnia. *Sleep,* 22(8): 1–5.

Clayton MF. (2006). Communication: An important part of nursing care. *American Journal of Nursing,* 106: 70–71.

Cole C & Richards K. (2007). Sleep disruption in older adults. *American Journal of Nursing,* 107(5): 40–49.

Coulehan JL & Block MR. (1999). *The Medical Interview: Mastering Skills for Clinical Practice.* Philadelphia: F.A. Davis, p. 148.

Eskreis TR. (1998). Seven common legal pitfalls in nursing. *American Journal of Nursing,* 98(4): 34–40.

Foreman MD, et al. (2003). Assessing cognitive function. In Mezey M, et al. (Eds.). *Geriatric Nursing Protocols for Best Practice,* 2nd ed. New York: Springer, pp. 99–115.

Glass RD. (1996). *Diagnosis: A Brief Introduction.* New York: Oxford University Press.

Gordon M. (1992). High-risk nursing diagnoses in critical care. In Carroll-Johnson, R. (Ed.). *Classification of Nursing Diagnoses: Proceedings of the Tenth Conference.* Philadelphia: Lippincott.

Gordon M. (2007). *Manual of Nursing Diagnoses,* 10th ed. St. Louis: Mosby.

Gordon M. (2007). *Nursing Diagnosis: Process and Application.* St. Louis: Mosby-Elsevier. Functional Health Patterns, Chapters 4–6.

Gordon M. (1994). *Nursing Diagnosis: Process and Application,* 3rd ed. St. Louis: Mosby.

Gordon M. (1996). Report of an RNF study: Diagnostic criteria for selected rehabilitation nursing diagnoses. *Rehabilitation Nursing Research,* 5: 1–6.

Gordon M. (1995). RNF project on high-frequency/high-treatment priority nursing diagnoses in rehabilitation nursing, part I. *Rehabilitation Nursing Research,* 4: 3–10.

Gordon M. (1995). RNF project on high-frequency/high-treatment priority nursing diagnoses in rehabilitation nursing, part II. *Rehabilitation Nursing Research,* 5: 38–46.

Gordon M & Murphy CM. (1994). Clinical judgment: An integrated model. *Advances in Nursing Science,* 16: 55–70.

Grace PJ. (2004). Patient safety and the limits of confidentiality. *American Journal of Nursing,* 104(11): 33.

Harkreader, H. (2004). *Fundamentals of Nursing: Caring and Clinical Judgment.* St. Louis: Saunders-Elsevier.

Hodgson IA. (1991). Why do we need sleep? Relating theory to nursing practice. *Journal of Advanced Nursing,* 16(12): 1503–1510.

Johns M. (1991). Epworth sleepiness scale. *Sleep,* 14(6): 540–545.

Jones D. (2002). Establishing the psychometic properties of the FHPAST: Use in practice. *Journal of Japan Society of Nursing*, 7(1): 12–17.

Jones D (1986). Health assessment manual. St. Louis: McGraw-Hill.

Katz A. (2006). Erectile dysfunction and its discontents. *American Journal of Nursing*, 106(12): 70–72.

Keefe S. (2006). Post-acute rehab: A delicate matter. *Nursing Advance, New England*, November 20, 2006, pp. 25–28, www.advanceweb.com

Morris JN, et al. (1990). Designing the National Resident Assessment Instrument for nursing homes. *The Gerontologist*, 30: 293–307.

McCaffery, et al. (2004). Prayer for health concerns: Results of a national survey on prevalence and patterns of use. *Archives of Internal Medicine*, April 26(4).

McCourt, AE (Ed.). (1993). *The Specialty Practice of Rehabilitation Nursing: A Core Curriculum*, 3rd ed. Skokie, Ill.: Rehabilitation Nursing Foundation, p. 108.

NANDA International. (2007). *Nursing Diagnoses: Definitions and Classification, 2007–2008*. Philadelphia: Author.

St. Romain, P. (1993). *Handbook for Spiritual Growth*. Liguori, Mo.: Liguori Publications.

Schumacher K, et al. (2006). Family caregivers. *American Journal of Nursing*, 106(8): 40–49.

Welker-Hood K. (2006). Does workplace stress lead to accident or error? *American Journal of Nursing*, 106(9): 104.

Wyman JF, et al. (Eds.). (2004). Shaping future directions for incontinence research: Reports from an international nursing summit. *Nursing Research*, Supplement to November/December 53(6S): S1–S59.

Reviewers

Index

Note: Page numbers followed by f refer to figures (illustrations).